The Guru Method

Organic Chemistry

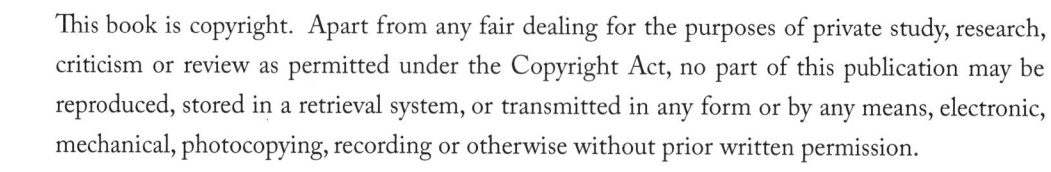

This book is copyright. Apart from any fair dealing for the purposes of private study, research, criticism or review as permitted under the Copyright Act, no part of this publication may be reproduced, stored in a retrieval system, or transmitted in any form or by any means, electronic, mechanical, photocopying, recording or otherwise without prior written permission.

For information contact:

GSMS Education Pty Ltd
P.O Box 3848
Marsfield NSW
2122
Australia

Organic Chemistry - The Guru Method

Organic Chemistry is part of the 40% of chemistry that will be represented in the GAMSAT exam. It is generally assumed that chemistry is the most difficult part of Section III. If you learn the method for answering these questions, you will find that studying for organic chemistry is less of an "information overload" than you may think. It is recommended that you work your way through the "General Chemistry" guide first to get an understanding of chemistry.

This manual is arranged exactly the same as the General Chemistry manual. It starts out with some basic facts, followed by practice problems, and finally the GAMSAT style questions.

The most important part of this manual is Chapter 3: Reaction Types. Nearly every single year, questions from this topic appear in the GAMSAT Section III exam. Students coming across these questions will panic if they are not familiar with the so-called "reaction mechanism". These questions boil down to recognizing patterns. This manual will prepare you well. The Reaction Types topic can represent a significant portion of the organic chemistry questions in the GAMSAT.

Table of Contents

Organic Chemistry - The Guru Method 3

CHAPTER 1: Nomenclature and Physical Properties 5
    Key Concepts: Chemical Bonding 5
    Key Concepts: Inter-molecular Forces 5
    Key Concepts: Nomenclature and Structural Theory 6
    Quick Facts: Hydrocarbons 7
    Quick Facts: Alkanes 8
    Key Concepts: Alkanes 10
    Quick Facts: Alkenes 10
    Key Concepts: Alkenes 10
    Quick Facts: Alkynes 11
    Key Concepts: Alkynes 11
    Quick Facts: Trends in the Solubility of Hydrocarbons 11
    Quick Facts: Trends in Melting and Boiling points of Hydrocarbons 12
    Quick Facts: Carbocations and Stabilization 12
    Practice Questions 13
    GAMSAT Style Questions 26

CHAPTER 2: Strength of Carboxylic Acids and Amines 33
    Key Concepts: Carboxylic Acids 33
    Key Concepts: Acid Strength 34
    Quick Facts: Basicity of Amines 36
    Key Concept: Resonance Effect 37
    GAMSAT Style Questions 38

CHAPTER 3: Reaction Types: The GAMSAT Chemistry Challenge ... 51
    Illustrative Questions 55
    GAMSAT Style Questions 57

CHAPTER 4: Isomerism 93
    Key Concept: Isomerism 93
    Key Concepts: Structural Isomerism 93
    Key Concept: Stereoisomerism 96
    Quick Facts: Geometrical Isomerism 96
    Key Concept: Optical Isomerism 96
    Quick Facts: Optical Isomerism 97
    Practice Questions 98
    GAMSAT Style Questions 103

Chapter 1: **Nomenclature and Physical Properties**

> *Tip:* The "Key Concepts" sections are general principles that can be found in Organic Chemistry textbooks. We have provided them for your own "quick reference" and they are not intended to replace a textbook. If you do not understand any of the Key Concepts, you will need to gain an understanding of the topic by getting an Organic Chemistry textbook and studying from that until you are familiar with the concepts listed.

Key Concepts: Chemical Bonding

Organic chemistry is the chemistry of the compounds of carbon. In order to gain an understanding of the structure of molecules, one must first understand chemical bonds. The two main types of chemical bonds are *ionic bonds* and *covalent bonds*. Bonds occur via electrons in the outer or valence shell. All elements "want" a full valence shell.

1. Ionic bond: Results from the transfer of electrons. For example, in the formation of Lithium Fluoride, Li has one electron in its valence shell and F has 7. Therefore, Li transfers that one electron to the valence shell of F such that Li now has a positive charge and F acquires a negative charge. These opposite charges then attract each other.

2. Covalent bond: Results from the sharing of electrons. For example, the formation of a hydrogen molecule. Both H's have a single electron and thus by sharing those electrons, both molecules can fill their valence shells. This type of bond is typical of carbon compounds and thus the bond of chief importance in organic chemistry

Key Concepts: Inter-molecular Forces

The forces holding the molecules of non-ionic compounds are called *intermolecular forces*. There are two types of intermolecular forces, *dipole-dipole interactions and van der Waals forces*.
1. dipole-dipole interactions: attraction of the positive end of one polar molecule with the negative end of another polar molecule. *Hydrogen bonding* is the strongest type of dipole-dipole interaction, it occurs when H acts a bridge between two electronegative atoms holding one by a covalent bond and the other by purely electrostatic forces. For hydrogen bonding to occur, the electronegative atoms must be one of the following: F, O, N.
2. van der Waals forces: the attractive forces that occur between non-polar molecules. These types of forces are of particular importance in holding together hydrocarbon compounds.

Key Concepts: Nomenclature and Structural Theory

All organic compounds are separated into a number of families based on their chemical structure. By doing this, the compounds are at the same time classified as to their physical and chemical properties since a particular set of properties is characteristic of a particular structure. Of course, within each family, there will be variations in properties. i.e. One member of a family may react more readily with a particular reagent than others; however all will react with that reagent. In the quick facts section, we will provide you with a brief overview of the structure of the families important in the study of organic chemistry.

> ***Tip:*** **The Quick Facts section is designed to give you a PRACTICAL summary of important topics for the GAMSAT. It is not intended to be a full explanation of the topic. It is designed to give you the "straight dope" on what is required to answer the GAMSAT questions in this topic. The "Quick Facts" illustrates what is needed to understand GAMSAT questions and not be confused with the jargon that the GAMSAT regularly displays.**

--->Quick Facts: Hydrocarbons

1. Alkanes - only carbon and hydrogen and all single bonds.

2. Functional groups with C-C multiple bonds.

   a. Alkenes $\quad$ C=C

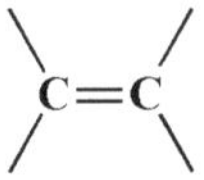

   b. Alkynes 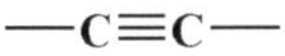 $\quad$ —C≡C—

   c. Arenes (benzene ring)

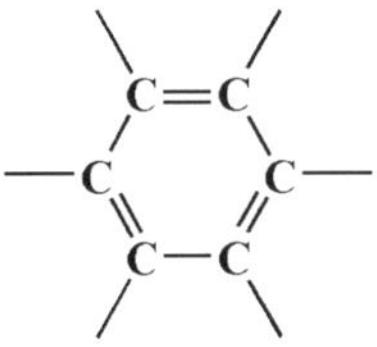

Carbon singly bonded to electronegative atoms

   1. Alcohols   R-OH
   2. Ethers   R-O-R`
   3. Amines   R-NH$_2$, R$_2$NH, R$_3$N
   4. Sulfides   R-S-R`
   5. Thiols   R-SH
   6. Other   sulfones, sulfoxides

Carbon doubly bonded to oxygen

1. Aldehydes

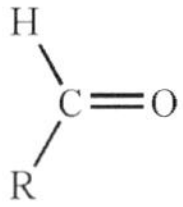

$$\begin{array}{c} H \\ \diagdown \\ C=O \\ \diagup \\ R \end{array}$$

2. Ketones

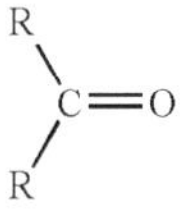

$$\begin{array}{c} R \\ \diagdown \\ C=O \\ \diagup \\ R \end{array}$$

3. Carboxylic Acids

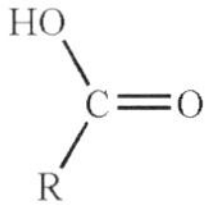

$$\begin{array}{c} HO \\ \diagdown \\ C=O \\ \diagup \\ R \end{array}$$

4. Ester

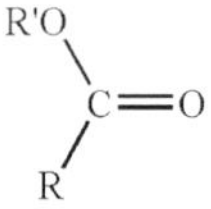

$$\begin{array}{c} R'O \\ \diagdown \\ C=O \\ \diagup \\ R \end{array}$$

5. Amide

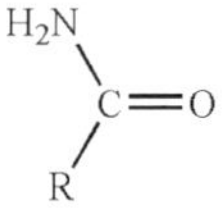

$$\begin{array}{c} H_2N \\ \diagdown \\ C=O \\ \diagup \\ R \end{array}$$

6. Acid halide

$$\begin{array}{c} X \\ \diagdown \\ C=O \\ \diagup \\ R \end{array}$$

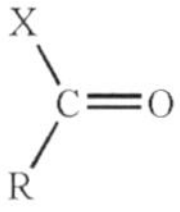

where R must be H or a hydrocarbon

-->*Quick Facts:* Alkanes

General Formula C_nH_{2n+2}

- Alkanes have only single bonds.
- The hybridization on carbon is sp^3.
- Carbon-carbon bonds are sp^3-sp^3 overlap to form sigma bonds.
- Carbon-hydrogen bonds are sp^3-s overlap to also form sigma bonds.

Chapter 1: Nomenclature and Physical Properties

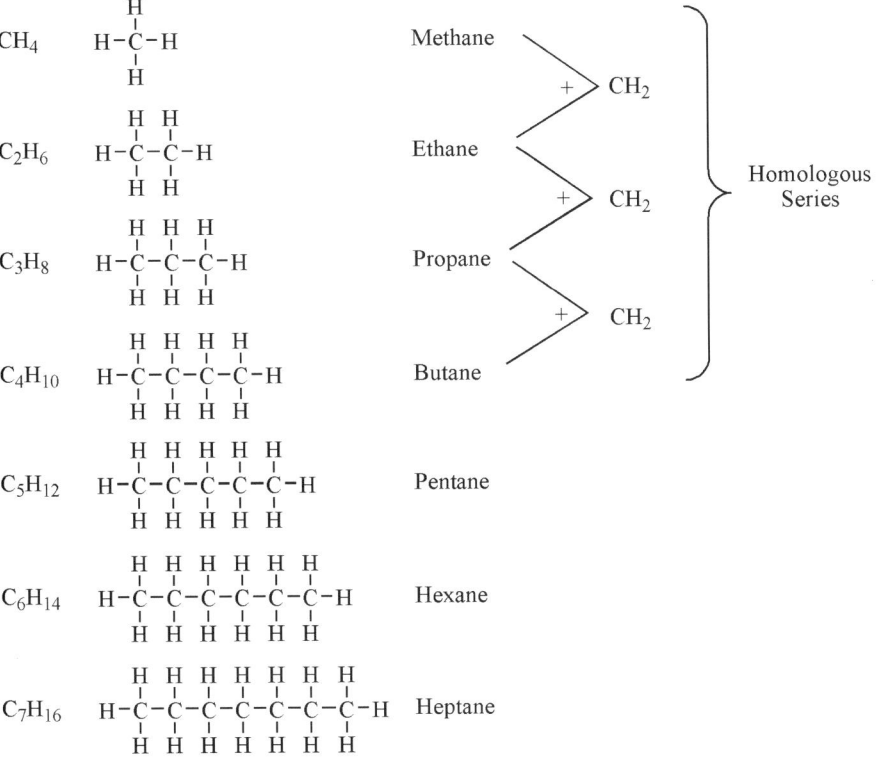

- If a hydrogen atom is removed from an alkane, what remains is an alkyl group. $CH_4 \rightarrow CH_3-$; The name of this group is a METHYL group.

Name	Group	Abbreviation	Example
CH_3-	Methyl	Me-	Methyl alcohol
CH_3CH_2-	Ethyl	Et-	Ethyl chloride
$CH_3CH_2CH_2-$	Propyl	Pr-	Propyl amine
$CH_3CH_2CH_2CH_2-$	Butyl	Bu-	Butyl bromide

Key Concepts: Alkanes

There is a regular increase in boiling point and melting with the increase in molecular weight when comparing the straight-chain homologous series.

Branching lowers boiling point when you compare compounds of same molecular weight (isomers). Pentane 36.1°C, isopentane 27.8°C, neopentane 9.5°C. Alkanes are non-polar compounds with only weak van der Waals attractions holding the molecules together. These forces only operate over small distances and are not uniform throughout the system. Temporary dipoles have a fleeting existence.

--->*Quick Facts:* Alkenes

- Almost identical to Alkanes of same Molecular Weight.
- Similar trends to alkanes with respect to melting and boiling points, can depend. on position of double bond.

Key Concepts: Alkenes

The physical properties of alkenes are essentially the same as those of alkanes. They are insoluble in water, and quite soluble in non-polar solvents. They are less dense than water, and like alkanes, the boiling point increases regularly with increasing carbon number. Their boiling points and melting points are almost identical to their alkane counterparts. Branching lowers the melting and boiling point of alkenes.

Like alkanes, alkenes are only weakly polar. The loosely held π electrons of the double bond are easily pulled or pushed, thus the dipole moments are larger than for alkanes albeit still small. An alkene with the *cis* configuration will have a small dipole, however in the case of the *trans* configuration, the bond moments on each side of the molecule cancel each other out and thus the dipole moment is 0. Because of its higher polarity, the *cis* isomer generally has the higher boiling point, and because of its lower symmetry it generally has the lower melting point (however, there are exceptions).

Chapter 1: Nomenclature and Physical Properties

-->Quick Facts: Alkynes

- Carbon—Carbon triple bonds.
- sp hybridized.
- Very short C≡C bond distance, much shorter than the C=C and the C—C distance.
- Almost identical to Alkanes/Alkenes of same Molecular Weight.
- Similar trends to alkanes with respect to melting and boiling points, can depend on position of double bond.

Key Concepts: Alkynes

The physical properties of alkynes are essentially the same as those of alkanes and alkenes. They show the same behaviour with respect to solubility, density, melting, and boiling points. Branching lowers the melting and boiling point. Similar to alkenes, alkynes have weakly held π electrons and therefore possess a small dipole moment.

-->Quick Facts: Trends in the Solubility of Hydrocarbons

> **Tip:** Given below is a detailed description of the solubility of hydrocarbons as they increase in the number of carbon atoms they contain, there is no need to remember the specific numbers but be aware of the trends in this information.

A. Hydrocarbon Series - Alkanes

Alkane	# C atoms	S_w, mg/L
n-butane	4	61
n-pentane	5	40
n-hexane	6	12
n-heptane	7	6
Hexadecane	16	0.0009
Iso-pentane	5	49
2,2-Dimethylbutane	6	20
Cyclohexane	6	60

Trends: a. ↑ # C atoms, ↓ water solubility
b. branching ↑ water solubility (for equivalent # C atoms)
c. aromatics ↑ water solubility (for equivalent # C atoms)

B. Hydrocarbon Series - Alkenes & Alkynes

Compound	# C atoms	S_w, mg/L	S_w, Ref.
2-hexene, Me-C=C-Pr	6	78	12
1,4-pendadiene, H_2C=C-C-C=CH_2	5	558	40
1-pentyne, C≡C-Pr	5	1570	40
benzene, C_6H_6	6	1770	12

Trends: unsaturation ↑ S_w, proportional to number of multiple bonds

C. Aryl Halides (C_6)

Compound	# Cl atoms	S_w, mg/L	S_w, Ref.
Chlorobenzene	1	500	1770
p-dichlorobenzene	2	85	"
Pentachlorobenzene	5	0.56	"
Hexachlorobenzene	6	0.005	"

Trends: ↓ S_w, proportional to number of Cl atoms bonded

--->Quick Facts: Trends in Melting and Boiling points of Hydrocarbons

- M.p. and B.p. increase with increasing molecular weight.
- Solubility decreases with increasing molecular weight for equivalent numbers of carbons.
- M.p. and B.p. decrease with branching.
- Solubility increases with branching, cyclization, and unsaturation.

--->Quick Facts: Carbocations and Stabilization

A carbocation is a molecule in which a carbon atom bears three bonds and a positive charge. The stability of a carbocation is dependant on a few factors:

- Resonance: A stabilizing factor because delocalizes the positive charge and creates additional bonding between adjacent atoms. In general, any adjacent lone pairs of electrons or π bond can be involved in resonance delocalization.
- Inductive effect: This results in the dispersal of charge, where the electron density of the sigma bonds is shifted toward the positive carbon. This shift creates a partial positive charge on the adjacent atoms, thus the positive charge is somewhat dispersed. Alky groups contain more atoms and electrons than an H.
- Hyperconjugative effect: In this case, bonding electrons from neighboring sigma bonds may overlap with the unoccupied p orbital of the carbocation. This overlap provides electron density to the electron deficient carbocation. Thus, the more bonds attached to the positive carbon results in an increase in stability, although only C-H and C-C bonds provide a significant level of increased stability.
- For carbocation stability the following applies:
    - Methyl < 1° < 2° < 3°

Tip: Practise questions are designed so that they test your understanding of the topic, they are not GAMSAT style questions in that they do not provide you with the information needed to answer the questions.

Practice Questions

Questions (1 – 5).

The only attractive forces in alkanes are weak van der Waals forces. Owing to its large surface area, the van der Walls attractive forces are relatively large. The greater the branching, the lower the surface area. The more intermolecular forces between the molecules in a compound the higher the boiling point.

1. Which of the following compound has the highest boiling point?
    A. n-hexane
    B. n-pentane
    C. 2, 2-dimethyl propane
    D. 2-methyl butane

2. The highest boiling point is expected for
    A. Iso octane
    B. n-octane
    C. 2, 2, 3, 3-tetramethyl butane
    D. n-butane

3. Which of the following isomer of pentane has the lowest boiling point?
    A. n-pentane
    B. neo pentane
    C. iso-pentane
    D. all have the same

4. Which one of the following is expected to have high volatility?
    A. n-butane
    B. n-pentane
    C. 2-methyl butane
    D. 2,2-dimethyl propane

5. Which of the following statement is NOT correct regarding alkanes?
    A. The alkanes are almost insoluble in water, but readily soluble in ether.
    B. The density of the normal alkanes increases down the homologous series.
    C. The melting point of the normal alkanes decreases down the series with increases in molecular mass.
    D. The normal alkane always has the higher boiling point than the branched alkane.

Questions (6-7).

6. The correct order of ease of substitution of hydrogen is
    A. 3° > 1° > 2°
    B. 3° > 2° < 1°
    C. 3° > 2° > 1°
    D. 3° < 1° > 2°

7. The order of reactivity of halogen towards halogenation of alkanes is
    A. $F_2 > Br_2 > Cl_2$
    B. $F_2 > Cl_2 > Br_2$
    C. $Cl_2 > F_2 > Br_2$
    D. $Cl_2 < Br_2 > F_2$

Chapter 1: Nomenclature and Physical Properties

Question (8 – 9).

8. The order of stability of alkenes $R_2C = CR_2$, $R_2C = CHR$ and $RCH = CHR$ is
   A. $RCH = CHR > R_2C = CHR > R_2C = CR_2$
   B. $RCH = CHR < R_2C = CHR > R_2C = CR_2$
   C. $RCH = CHR > R_2C = CHR < R_2C = CR_2$
   D. $RCH = CHR < R_2C = CHR < R_2C = CR_2$

9. The order of stability of the carbonium ion is 3° > 2° > 1°
   The rate of addition of HX across the double bond in
   $(CH_3)_2 C = CH_2$, $CH_3CH = CH_2$ and $CH_2 = CH_2$ follows the order
   A. $(CH_3)_2 C = CH_2 > CH_3CH = CH_2 > CH_2 = CH_2$
   B. $(CH_3)_2 C = CH_2 < CH_3CH = CH_2 < CH_2 = CH_2$
   C. $(CH_3)_2 C = CH_2 < CH_3CH = CH_2 > CH_2 = CH_2$
   D. $(CH_3)_2 C = CH_2 > CH_3CH = CH_2 < CH_2 = CH_2$

Questions (10- 15).

10. The product 'X' in the following reaction is

$H_3CHC=CHCH_3 \xrightarrow{H_2O_2} 'X_1' \xrightarrow{HIO_4} 2X$

A. $CH_3-\underset{OH}{CH}-\underset{OH}{CH}-CH_3$

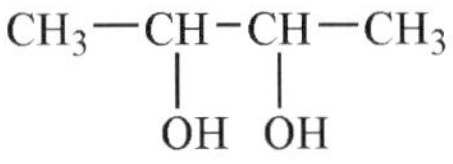

B. CH_3COOH

C. CH_3CHO

D. $H_3C-\underset{OH}{CH}-\underset{O}{\overset{\|}{C}}-CH_3$

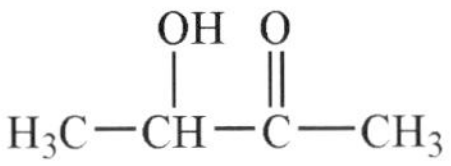

11. The product 'A' is

$\underset{H_3C}{\overset{H_3C}{\diagdown}}C=CH_2 \xrightarrow[KMnO_4/KOH]{Cold} A \xrightarrow[H_2SO_4]{K_2Cr_2O_7} \underset{H_3C}{\overset{H_3C}{\diagdown}}C=O + \underset{H-\overset{\|}{C}=O}{OH} + H_2O$

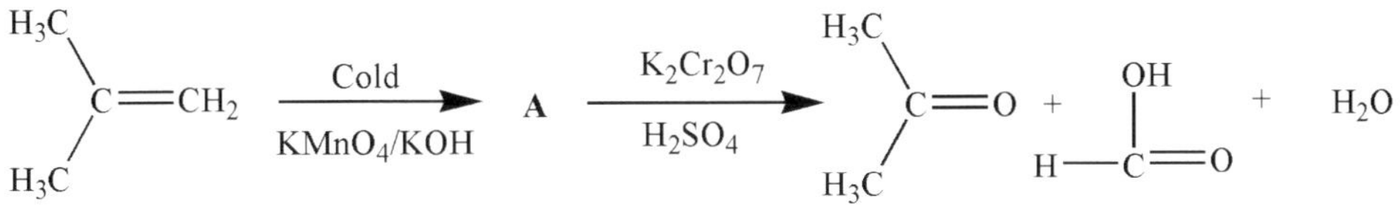

A. 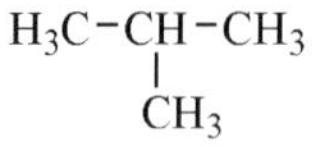 H₃C-CH-CH₃
         |
         CH₃

B. 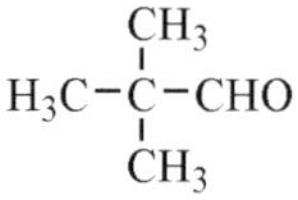 H₃C-C(CH₃)(CH₃)-CHO

C. H₃C-C(OH)(CH₃)-COOH

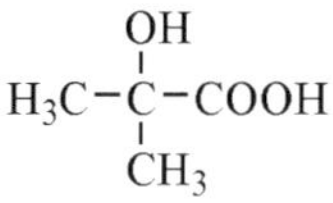

D. 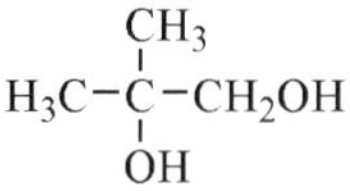 H₃C-C(CH₃)(OH)-CH₂OH

12. Acetylenic hydrogen is acidic because
    A. Sigma electron density of C – H bond in acetylene is nearer a carbon which has 50% s-character.
    B. Acetylene has only one hydrogen atom at each carbon atom
    C. Acetylene contains least number of hydrogen atoms among the possible hydrocarbons.
    D. Acetylene belongs to the class of alkynes with formula C_nH_{2n-2}

13. Which of the following has the shortest carbon-carbon bond length?
    A. C_2H_5OH
    B. C_2H_2
    C. C_2H_6
    D. C_2H_4

14. Which of the following orders regarding acid strength is correct?
    A. $CH_3COOH > CH_3CH_2OH > HC \equiv CH$
    B. $CH_3COOH > HC \equiv CH > CH_3CH_2OH$
    C. $HC \equiv CH > CH_3COOH > CH_3CH_2OH$
    D. $HC \equiv CH > CH_3CH_2OH > CH_3COOH$

15. Which of the following orders regarding base strength is correct?
    A. $CH_3COO^- > CH_3CH_2O^- < HC \equiv C^-$
    B. $HC \equiv C^- > CH_3COO^- > CH_3CH_2O^-$
    C. $HC \equiv C^- > CH_3CH_2O^- > CH_3COO^-$
    D. $CH_3COO^- > HC \equiv C^- > CH_3CH_2O^-$

Questions (16 – 19).

16. Consider the following reactions
    $RONa + H_2O \rightarrow ROH + NaOH$
    $NaNH_2 + ROH \rightarrow NaOR + NH_3$

    According to the above equations, which of the following orders regarding base strength is correct?
    A. $OH^- < NH_2^- < RO^-$
    B. $NH_2^- < OH^- < RO^-$
    C. $OH^- < RO^- < NH_2^-$
    D. $RO^- < NH_2^- < OH^-$

17. The relative stability order of carbanions $CH \equiv C^-$, CH_3^- and $CH_2 = CH^-$ is:
    A. $CH \equiv C^- > CH_2 = CH^- > CH_3^-$
    B. $CH_2 = CH^- > CH_3^- > CH \equiv C^-$
    C. $CH_3^- > CH_2 = CH^- > CH \equiv C^-$
    D. $CH \equiv C^- > CH_3^- > CH_2 = CH^-$

18. The relative stability order of stability of carbocations:

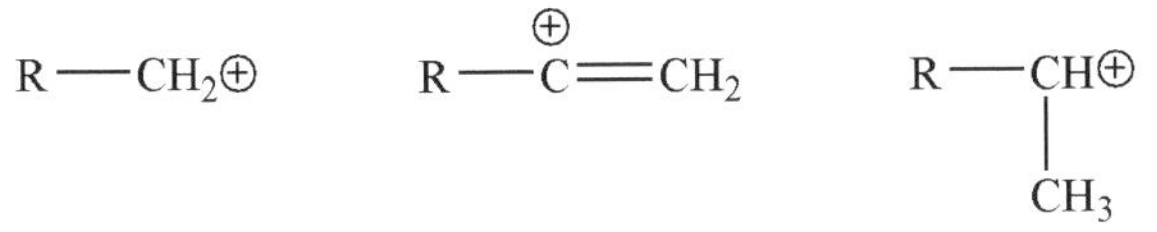

    $R-CH_2^\oplus \qquad R-\overset{\oplus}{C}=CH_2 \qquad R-\underset{\underset{CH_3}{|}}{CH^\oplus}$

A. 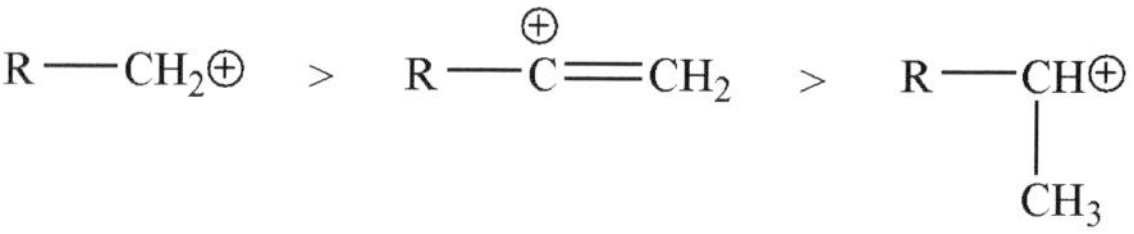 R—CH$_2^⊕$ > R—C$^⊕$=CH$_2$ > R—CH$^⊕$—CH$_3$

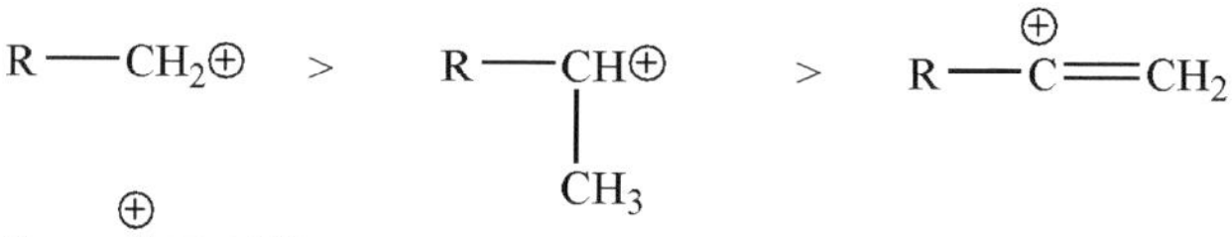

B. R—CH$_2^⊕$ > R—CH$^⊕$—CH$_3$ > R—C$^⊕$=CH$_2$

C. R—C$^⊕$=CH$_2$ > R—CH$_2^⊕$ > R—CH$^⊕$—CH$_3$

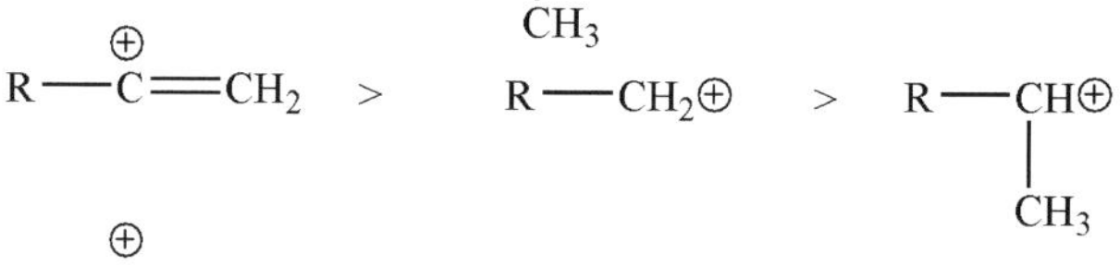

D. 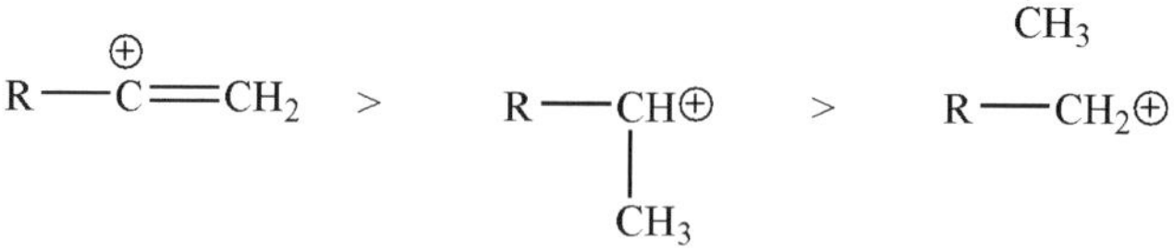 R—C$^⊕$=CH$_2$ > R—CH$^⊕$—CH$_3$ > R—CH$_2^⊕$

19. Which of the following carbocations is expected to be most stable?

A.

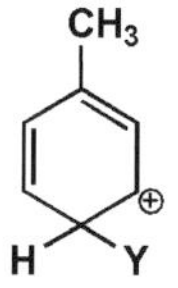

B.

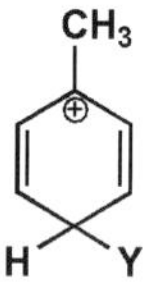

C.

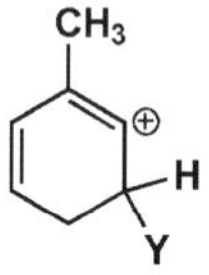

D.

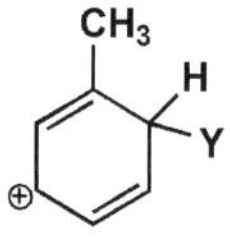

Question (20 – 21).

A compound is more stable if each atom has a complete octet.

20. Which of the following statement is correct?

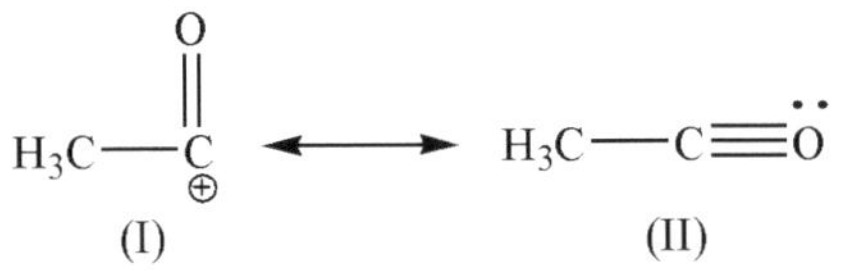

$$H_3C-\underset{(I)}{\overset{O}{\underset{\oplus}{C}}} \quad \longleftrightarrow \quad \underset{(II)}{H_3C-C\equiv\overset{..}{O}}$$

A. I is more stable than II
B. II is less stable than I because a positive charge is present on the more electronegative oxygen
C. II is more stable than I due to the presence of triple bond
D. II is more stable than I because each atom has eight electrons in its valence shell

21. The correct order of activating power of a group in benzene is
A. —NH$_2$ > —NHCOCH$_3$ > —CH$_3$
B. —NH$_2$ < —NHCOCH$_3$ < —CH$_3$
C. —NH$_2$ > —NHCOCH$_3$ < —CH$_3$
D. —NH$_2$ < —NHCOCH$_3$ > —CH$_3$

Solutions

Question 1

The only attractive forces in alkanes are weak van der Waals forces. In a group of isomeric compounds, the normal compound always have the highest b.p, and generally, the greater the branching, the lower is the b.p. n – hexane will have the highest b.p. answer A. Owing to its large surface area, the van der Walls attractive forces are relatively large.

Question 2

The answer is B. Due to linear structure and large surface area, it has a higher b.p.

Question 3

The greater the branching, the lower the surface area, the lower is the b.p. Out of three isomers of pentane, neopentane is highly branched and has a smallest surface area, lowest b.p. the answer is B.

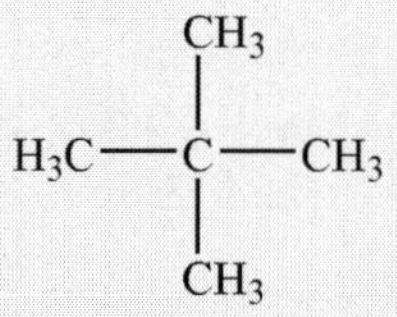

$$H_3C-\underset{\underset{CH_3}{|}}{\overset{\overset{CH_3}{|}}{C}}-CH_3 \qquad CH_3CH_2CH_2CH_2CH_3$$

$$\text{Lowest b.p} \qquad\qquad \text{Highest b.p.}$$

Question 4

Volatility and the boiling point are inversely related. 2, 2-dimethyl propane, due to high branching, has a lowest boiling point, so it is highly volatile. The answer is D.

Question 5

The b.p. and the m.p. of alkanes increases down the homologous series because, the area of contact between the neighbouring molecules increases. Therefore, the incorrect statement is one given in answer C.

Question 6
The stability order of free radicals is

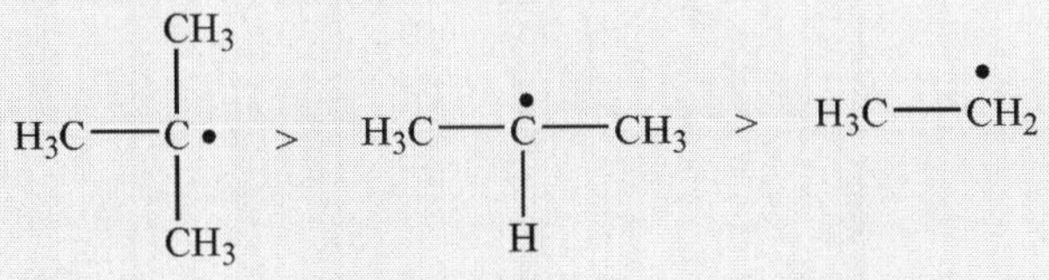

$$H_3C-\underset{\underset{CH_3}{|}}{\overset{\overset{CH_3}{|}}{C}}\cdot \quad > \quad H_3C-\overset{\cdot}{\underset{\underset{H}{|}}{C}}-CH_3 \quad > \quad H_3C-\overset{\cdot}{C}H_2$$

Replacement of H also follows this order, since a more stable structure will be more willing exchange H. This is because alkyl groups are weakly electron donating due to hyperconjugation and inductive effect. Resonance effect can further stabilise carbocation when present. So more stable 3° carbocation is highly reactive.
The answer is C.

Question 7
The order of reactivity of halogen for a give alkane follows the order

$$F_2 > Cl_2 > Br_2$$

Reactivity is dependant on the electronegativity of the molecule. The higher the electronegativity, the greater the attraction the molecule will have for bonding electrons. In the case on the halogens, the electronegativity decreases with increasing atomic number because the electrons are further away from the nucleus. Thus, the answer is B.

Question 8
As the number of alkyl groups in an alkene increases, hyper conjugation increases. Hyper conjugation stabilizes the alkene. The more hyper conjugation, the more stable the alkene. The correct order of stability is given in answer D.

Question 9
The more stable the carbonium ion the faster the addition of HX will be. Since the order of stability of the carbonium ion is 3° > 2° > 1°. The rate of addition of HX will follow the order $(CH_3)_2 C == CH_2 > CH_3CH == CH_2 > CH_2 == CH_2$ and this is given in answer A.

Question 10

The product 'X' is ethanal, CH_3CHO, answer C.
This is a method to determine the position of the double bond in the alkene.

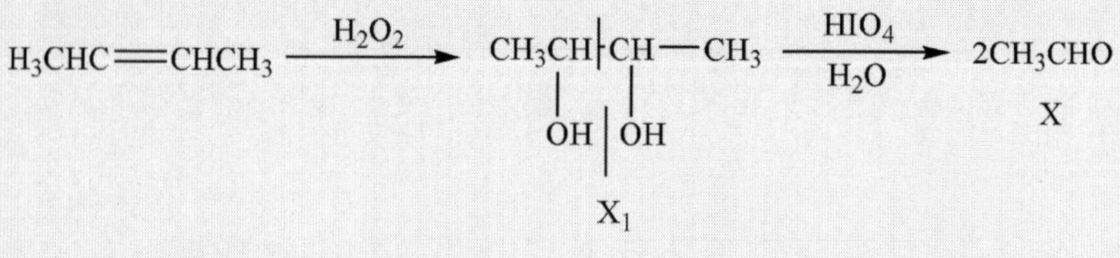

$$H_3CHC=CHCH_3 \xrightarrow{H_2O_2} CH_3CH(OH)-CH(OH)-CH_3 \xrightarrow[H_2O]{HIO_4} 2CH_3CHO$$

$$X_1 \qquad\qquad X$$

Question 11

Cold, alkaline potassium permanganate converts alkenes into cis-1,2-diols. Then, it reacts with the KOH as follows

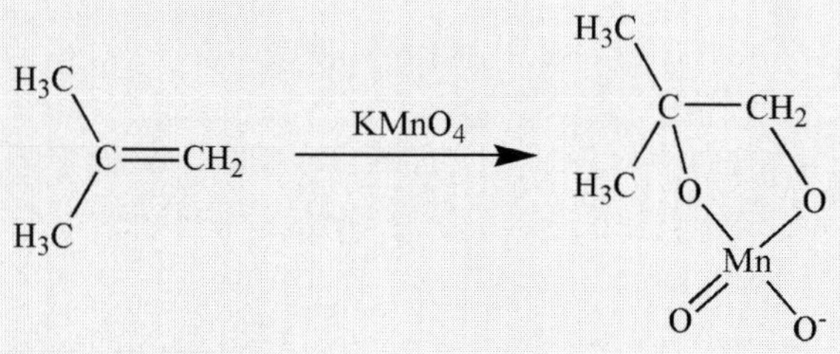

$$\underset{H_3C}{\overset{H_3C}{>}}C=CH_2 \xrightarrow{KMnO_4} \text{(cyclic manganate ester of } (CH_3)_2C\text{-}CH_2\text{ with } MnO_2^-\text{)}$$

The role of KOH is to keep the condition basic because in acidic conditions the diol is further oxidised. In this reaction, the manganate ester is rapidly hydrolyzed under the reaction conditions to yield the diol without the need for the reduction step and both oxygens originate on the MnO_4.

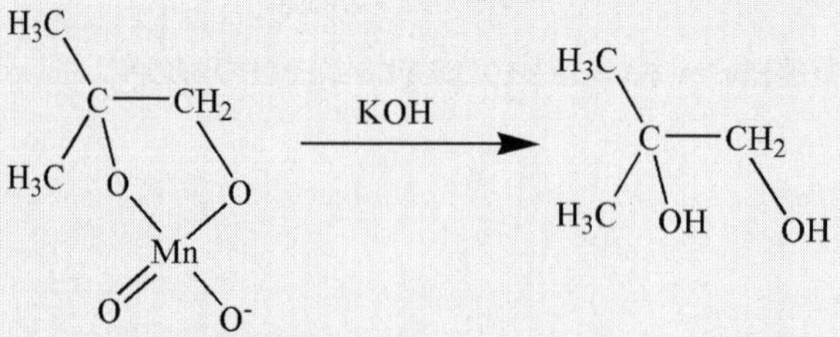

$$\text{(manganate ester)} \xrightarrow{KOH} \underset{H_3C}{\overset{H_3C}{>}}\underset{OH}{C}-\underset{OH}{CH_2}$$

So, compound A is cis-2-methyl-1,2-propandiol. Name of the final products are acetone and formic acid.

$$A \longrightarrow H_3C-\underset{CH_3}{\overset{OH}{C}}-CH_2OH$$

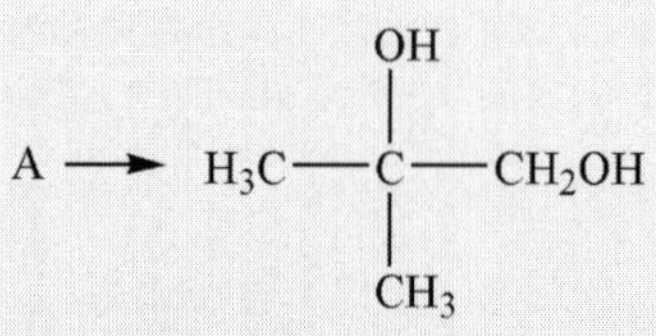

The answer is D.

Chapter 1: Nomenclature and Physical Properties

Question 12
The hybridization of C in acetylene is sp. sp carbons form two π bonds and have 50% s character. This sp carbon is more electronegative than sp². Thus, the sp C has more attraction for the electron and releases the proton easily. The answer is A.

Question 13
Bond length is inversely proportional to the number of bonds between the carbon atoms. In ethyne, there are three covalent bonds present between the carbon and carbon, so the bond length is the shortest. The answer is B.

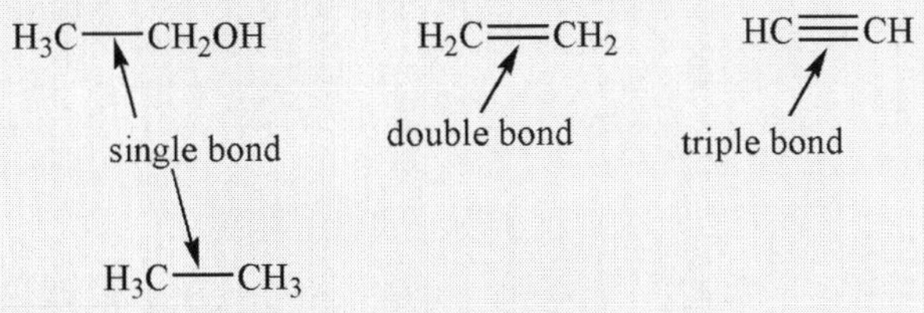

$H_3C\text{—}CH_2OH$ $H_2C\text{=}CH_2$ $HC\equiv CH$
single bond   double bond   triple bond

$H_3C\text{—}CH_3$

Question 14
The correct order of acidic strength is given in answer A. Remember acids donate protons. Thus, the molecule must be able to accommodate the electron pair left behind. An atom's electronegativity and size both contribute to its ability to accommodate an electron pair. Of the three molecules, CH_3COOH will be most able to accommodate the loss of the proton. The presence of the two oxygen molecules one having a double bond contributes to its ability to act as an acid. The double-bonded O will help to stabilize the anion due to resonance stabilization. The CH_3CH_2OH will be more acidic than $HC \equiv CH$ due to the presence of O since it is more electronegative than C.

Question 15
According to Bronsted – Lowry theory, weak acid has a strong conjugate base and strong acid has weak conjugate base. The acidic strength order of their parent acid (see solution #17).

   $CH_3COOH > CH_3CH_2OH > HC \equiv CH$
   Strongest acid   Weakest acid
The answer is C.

Question 16
The correct order is given in answer C.
As the reaction is more favoured in the forward direction, RO⁻ is a stronger base than OH⁻. On the basis of second reaction NH_2^- is stronger than RO⁻, as NH_2^- has formed NH_3. The correct order of basic strength therefore is OH⁻ < RO⁻ < NH_2^-

Question 17
The greater the electronegativity of an atom, the more readily it can accommodate a negative charge, the more stable the anion. A triple bond is more electronegative than a double bond, which is more than a single bond. The correct order of stability of carbanions is given in answer A.

Question 18
The stability of the carbocation depends on three main effects: resonance, inductive, and hyperconjugative. In most cases, resonance stabilisation will outweigh the effects of the other two.

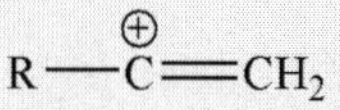

$R-\overset{\oplus}{C}=CH_2$ exhibits resonance stabilization through the π bond. In addition, the C-C and C-H bonds provides both hyperconjugation and induction. This is the most stable of the three

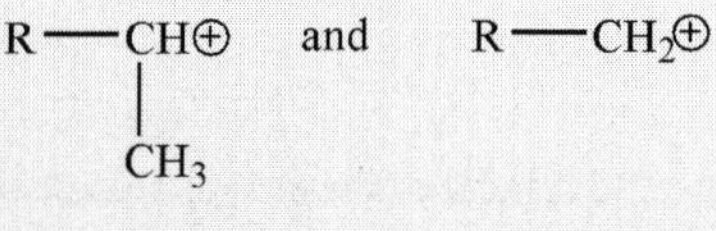

$$R-\overset{|}{\underset{CH_3}{C}H^\oplus} \quad \text{and} \quad R-CH_2^\oplus$$

do not exhibit resonance, but do exhibit the inductive effect and the hyperconjugative effect. However, the first molecule has an extra C-C bond and therefore, these effects will be stronger for this molecule making it more stable.

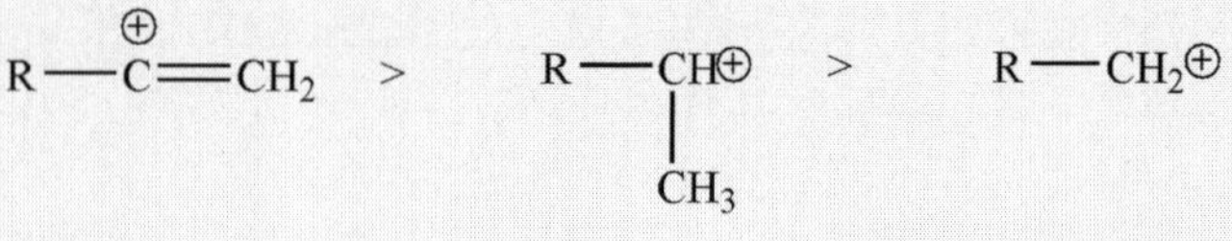

$$R-\overset{\oplus}{C}=CH_2 \quad > \quad R-\underset{CH_3}{\overset{|}{C}H^\oplus} \quad > \quad R-CH_2^\oplus$$

Therefore, the answer is D.

Question 19

The most stable carbocation is the one that is given in answer B, because the + charge is nearest to e- donating group. The e- group can help to neutralize the + charge and consequently this ion is stabilized.

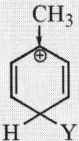

Question 20

The statement in answer D is correct
(II) is more stable than (I) because each atom has a complete octet.

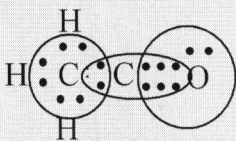

Question 21

The correct order is given in answer A.
— NH$_2$ group is the strongest activating group due to the presence of a lone pair of electrons on N. It has strong resonance effect (R). The CH$_3$ group is activating due to the inductive effect (I).

$$—NH_2 > —NHCOCH_3 > —CH_3$$
(+R effect)   (+ I effect)

GAMSAT Style Questions

> **Tip:** Our GAMSAT style questions will give you a gauge as to how you will perform in the actual GAMSAT. Try to pace yourself slightly faster than what you will have to achieve on the exam day. That is about 1 minute per question.

Question (1-6)

Consider a carbon chain in which one terminal carbon atom is joined to a more electronegative element (say Cl). —C_3—C_2—C_1—Cl. Cl has greater electronegativity than carbon therefore, the e- pair forming the covalent bond between C_1 and chlorine will be displaced towards the chlorine atom. This causes the Cl atom to acquire a small negative charge and C_1 a small positive charge, but the charge will be small on C_1 because the effect of the C_1 atom has been transmitted through C_1 to C_2. This type of electron displacement along a chain is known as the inductive effect, it is permanent, and decreases rapidly as the distance from the source increases. It is important to note that the electron pairs, although permanently displaced, remain in the same valency shells.

1. Which of the following statements can be inferred regarding the inductive effect?
    A. It implies the atom's ability to cause bond polarization
    B. It implies the transfer of a lone pair of electrons from the more electronegative atom in a molecule.
    C. It implies the transfer of a lone pair of electrons from the less electronegative atom to the more electronegative atom in a molecule.
    D. It increases with increasing in distance.

2. Each of the following group exerts a + I effect EXCEPT:
    A. $(CH_3)_3 C-$
    B. CO_2^-
    C. O^-
    D. OH

3. Which of the following group will not exert a + I effect?
   A. $(CH_3)_2 CH—$
   B. COO^-
   C. $CH_3—$
   D. $—NH_3^+$

4. Which of the following groups will exert a – I effect?
   A. $CH_3—$
   B. $C_6H_5^+—$
   C. $(CH_3)_2 CH—$
   D. CO_2^-

The resonance effect implies the dispersion of electrical charges over several atomic centres caused by the movement of delocalised electrons. This effect makes the species more stable. For example, the following carbanion gets stabilized due to resonance effect.

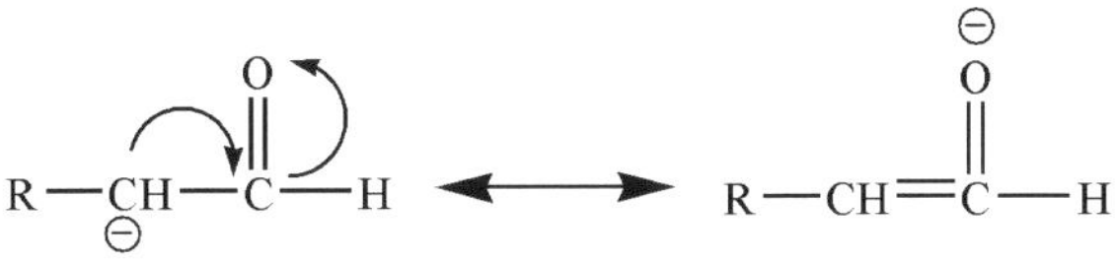

$$R—\overset{\ominus}{C}H—\overset{O}{\underset{}{C}}—H \longleftrightarrow R—CH=\overset{\overset{\ominus}{O}}{C}—H$$

A group that releases electrons to benzene ring is an activating group. A group that withdraws electrons from benzene is a deactivating group.

5. In which of the following molecules is the +R effect is present via the benzene ring?

A. 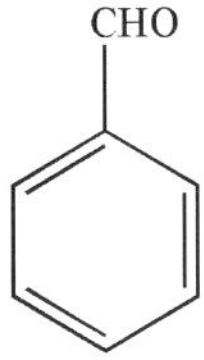 (benzene with CHO)   B. 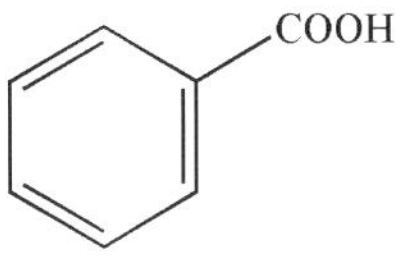 (benzene with COOH)   C. 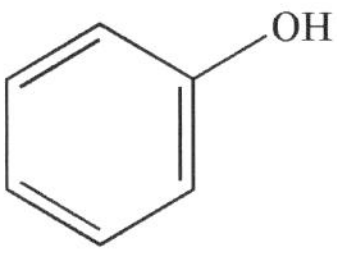 (benzene with OH)   D. 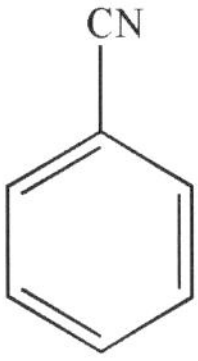 (benzene with CN)

6. Aniline is a weaker base than ethyl amine. This is due to

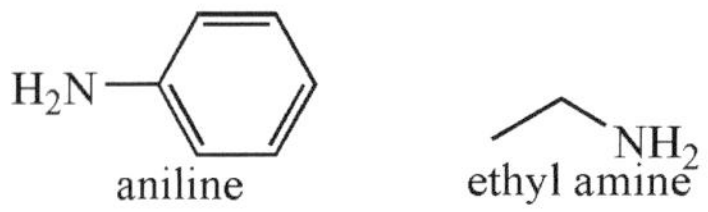

aniline

ethyl amine

A. − I effect of NH_2 in aniline
B. − R effect of NH_2 in aniline
C. + I effect of NH_2 in aniline
D. + R effect of NH_2 in aniline

Question 7
The following structures all have the same molecular formula: C_6H_{14}

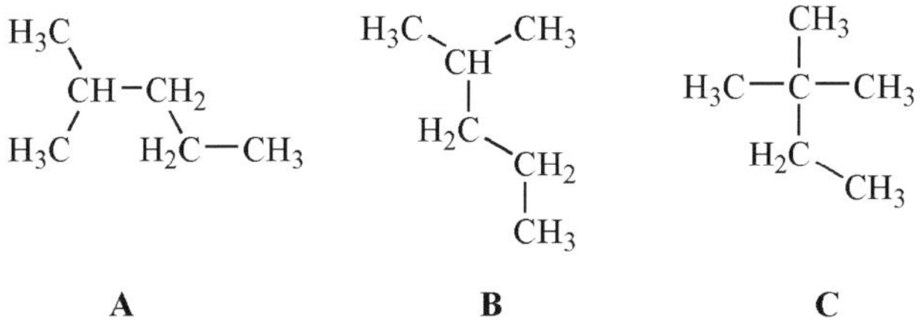

A

B

C

7. Which of these structures represent the same molecule?
   A. A and B
   B. B and C
   C. A and C
   D. None

Question 8
Combustion is an exothermic reaction.
8. Which of the following alkenes is the most stable?

Alkene	ΔH° Comb (kJ mol⁻¹)
A. $(CH_3)_2 C == CH_2$	- 2703
B. $CH_3CH_2CH == CH_2$	- 2719
C. cis $CH_3CH == CHCH_3$	- 2712
D. trans $CH_3CH == CHCH_3$	- 2707

Solution

> **Tip**: We introduce our three-step method to tackle any GAMSAT question. Step one is interpreting the question. This is a critical step because 90% of students who get the answer wrong in a GAMSAT question do so because they do not understand what the question is asking. Step two is analyzing the data. The third step is applying your knowledge to the given question.

Question 1.
STEP 1 = > <u>What do you need to determine to solve the problem?</u>
You need to determine the correct statement regarding the inductive effect.

STEP 2 = > <u>What relevant data provided in this problem is necessary in order to answer the question?</u>
The passage tells you that in a bond between carbon and an electronegative element such as Cl will result in the electronegative element acquiring a partial negative charge since it will attract the electrons in the bond towards itself. The carbon will acquire a partial positive charge because the electrons will be drawn away from it. The inductive effect will distribute this charge down the length of the chain, and the charge will decrease with distance from the Cl.

STEP 3 = > <u>Use the relevant data to solve the question</u>
The correct statement is one given in answer A. Due to the presence of an electronegative element (X), the C – X bond gets polarized.

$$\overset{\delta+\ \ \ \delta-}{-C_3-C_2-C_1 \rightarrow Cl}$$

It is important to note that the electron pairs, although permanently displaced, remain in the same valency shells.

Question 2.
STEP 1 = > <u>What do you need to determine to solve the problem?</u>
Which group does not exert a positive inductive effect.

STEP 2 = > <u>What relevant data provided in this problem is necessary in order to answer the question?</u>
You are told that the inductive effect is the ability of the carbon chain to distribute a partial positive charge throughout the chain. In this case you are dealing with the relative inductive effect.

STEP 3 => Use the relevant data to solve the question
A positive inductive effect is the ability of the group to release electrons to the rest of the molecule so that the effect can be distributed throughout the molecule. Therefore, any molecule that will not attract electrons towards itself but rather release them, will result in a +I effect. In contrast, a –I effect results from a group that withdraws electrons away from the rest of the molecule toward itself. Alkyl groups cause a +I effect because they are electron releasing. Choices B and C are anions and therefore being already negatively charge will not attract electrons to them, but rather release them to the rest of the molecule and therefore also have a +I effect. Because the OH group is electronegative, it will withdraw electrons towards itself from the rest of the molecule and therefore have a –I effect, so the answer is D.

Question 3.
STEP 1 => What do you need to determine to solve the problem?
Again, we are looking for which group does not exert a positive inductive effect.

STEP 2 => What relevant data provided in this problem is necessary in order to answer the question?
You are told that the inductive effect is the ability of the carbon chain to distribute a partial positive charge through the chain. Think of it as the molecules that will not attract the electron pair toward itself.

STEP 3 => Use the relevant data to solve the question
Due to positive charge, NH_3^+ will attract the electrons pair towards itself (it is electron withdrawing) and will exert a – I effect. The answer is D. The other three molecules are electron releasing in that they will release electrons to the rest of the chain to be distributed therefore they will have a +I effect.

Question 4.
STEP 1 => What do you need to determine to solve the problem?
You are now looking for the molecule that produces a negative inductive effect.

STEP 2 => What relevant data provided in this problem is necessary in order to answer the question?
You are told that the inductive effect is the ability of the carbon chain to distribute a partial positive charge through the chain. Therefore, a negative inductive effect will be the molecule that will attract the electron pair toward itself.

STEP 3 => Use the relevant data to solve the question
$C_6H_5^+$ - carries a positive charge on it and can attract the e^- density towards itself. This group will have a tendency to attract the electrons, so is e^- attracting and exerts a – I effect, answer is B.

Chapter 1: Nomenclature and Physical Properties

Question 5.

STEP 1 = > What do you need to determine to solve the problem?
You are looking for the molecule with the positive resonance effect.

STEP 2 = > What relevant data provided in this problem is necessary in order to answer the question?
You are told that the resonance effect is the ability of the molecule to distribute the electrical charge through the molecule via the movement of delocalised electrons. It shows that in a carbanion with a double bonded O group, the double bond will alternate with the C-O bond and the C-C bond of the negatively charged carbon

STEP 3 = > Use the relevant data to solve the question

In the compound given in answer C, the key atom is e⁻ rich, so exerts a + R effect
The other three molecules in the question will no exhibit resonance via the benzene ring because molecule A has an O double-bonded to the carbon attached to the ring. In order for resonance to occur, the double bond would have to shift between the C it is bonded to and the benzene ring. This is impossible because that would mean the C attached to the ring would end up with 5 bonds due to the shifting of the double bonds on the ring. The same problem would be encountered with molecule D which contains an N triple bonded to the C. In molecule B, the resonance would occur on the side group within the carboxyl group, but could not shift to the ring for the same reason as stated above.

Question 6.

STEP 1 = > What do you need to determine to solve the problem?
You need to determine why aniline is a weaker base than ethyl amine.

STEP 2 = > What relevant data provided in this problem is necessary in order to answer the question?
You should know that a base is a molecule that can accept a proton. You are looking for the molecule with the least partial positive charge and the greatest partial negative charge. In this case, you also need to consider resonance stabilization, as the question tells you it causes the distribution of negative charge throughout the molecule.

STEP 3 = > Use the relevant data to solve the question
The answer is D due to + R effect of NH_2 group. Recall, that basicity is the ability

to donate electrons. In this case, the N's in both compounds contain a lone pairs of electrons so both can act as bases. However, the strength of a base is determined by a number of factors including the ability of the molecule to distribute the electron density throughout itself thereby stabilizing the electron rich group (NH_2 in this case). Recall that resonance stabilization outweighs other forms of stabilization such as the inductive effect. In order for resonance stabilization to occur, you need the capability of delocalizing the negative charge, by shifting lone pairs of electrons and π bonds. Ethylamine does not exhibit this ability due to the lack of π bonds in the molecule; however, the benzene ring attached to the amine in aniline contains three π bonds. The lone pair can shift to create a resonance structure with a C=N double bond and two double bonds on the ring.

Question 7.
  STEP 1 = > What do you need to determine to solve the problem?
  Which molecules are the same from the given structures.

  STEP 2 = > What relevant data provided in this problem is necessary in order to answer the question?
  You are given 3 chemical structures with the same molecular formula.

  STEP 3 = > Use the relevant data to solve the question
  There is no difference between compounds A and B; they both contain a five-carbon chain with a branch on the second carbon. Compound C, on the other hand, contains a four-carbon chain with two branches on the second carbon atom. The correct answer is A.

Question 8.
Try your own 3-step method. Combustion is an exothermic reaction, therefore, the heats of combustion are all negative since heat is given off; The smaller ΔH is (numerically; i.e. absolute value), the more stable the alkene thus a smaller amount of heat is given off in the reaction. The alkene given in answer A is the most stable.

Chapter 2: Strength of Carboxylic Acids and Amines

Key Concepts: Carboxylic Acids

Of the organic compounds that possess significant acidity, the carboxylic acids are by far the most important. These compounds contain the carboxyl group:

Carboxyl group

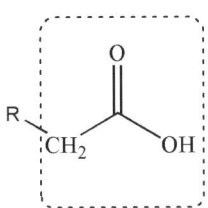

When naming carboxylic acids with common names, the greek letters are used to indicate the position of attachment. The α-carbon is the one bearing the carbonyl group, for instance:

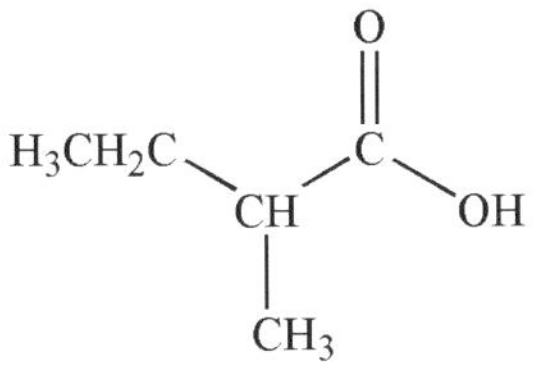

α-Methylbutyric acid

Also important to note, in IUPAC naming the substituents are numbered and the carboxyl carbon is always C_1, thus the α-carbon would be C_2.

Carboxylic acids are polar molecules and can form hydrogen bonds with each other and with other types of molecules. In terms of water solubility, the first 4 are miscible in water, the 5 carbon acid is partially miscible in water, and the higher carbon acids are insoluble in water. Carboxylic acids have fairly high boiling points, i.e. propionic acid boils at 141 °C, indicating that they are held together by two hydrogen bonds.

Key Concepts: Acid Strength

According to Bronsted-Lowry definition, an acid is a proton donor. The strength of an acid depends upon the ease with which an acid ionizes to give proton. Any atom or group that decreases the e⁻ density around H of COOH group helps in removing the H⁺ more easily. This increases the acid strength.

1) An electron-withdrawing group (-I group) attached to the carboxyl group withdraws e⁻ density inductively and decreases the e⁻ density around H thereby facilitating its release as H⁺. Therefore chloroacetic acid is stronger than acetic acid.

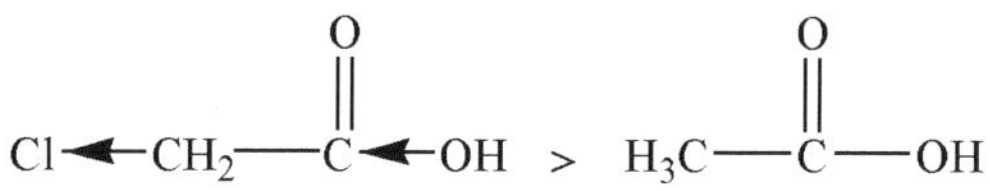

$$Cl \leftarrow CH_2 - C(=O) \leftarrow OH \quad > \quad H_3C - C(=O) - OH$$

$$pK_a = 2.82 \qquad\qquad pK_a = 4.72$$

2) The greater the number of -I groups present, the greater strength of the acid.

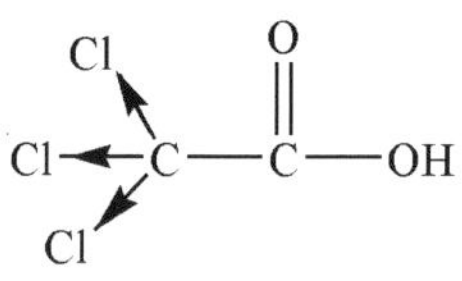

$$Cl_3C - C(=O) - OH \qquad Cl_2CH - C(=O) - OH \qquad Cl - CH_2 - C(=O) - OH$$

$$pK_a = 0.64 \qquad pK_a = 1.26 \qquad pK_a = 2.85$$

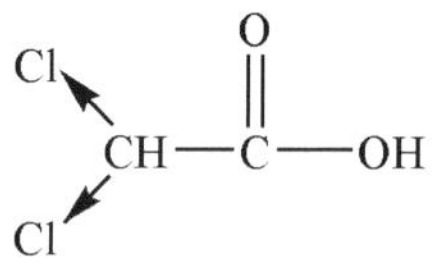

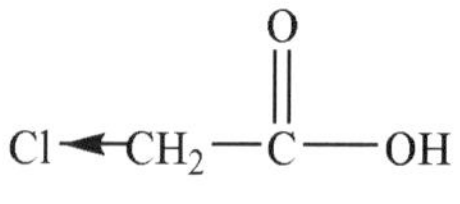

3) The greater the electronegativity of the halogen atom, the greater the strength of the acid.

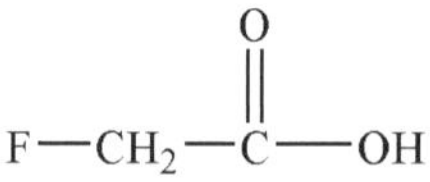

$$F - CH_2 - C(=O) - OH \qquad Cl - CH_2 - C(=O) - OH \qquad Br - CH_2 - C(=O) - OH$$

$$pK_a = 2.66 \qquad pK_a = 2.85 \qquad pK_a = 2.90$$

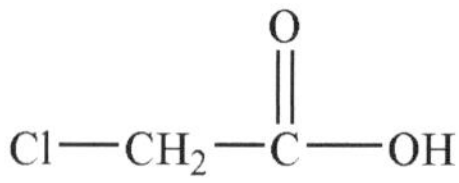

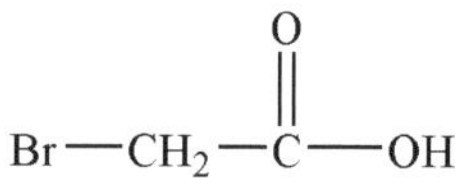

Chapter 2: Strength of Carboxylic Acids and Amines

4) Since the inductive effect decreases rapidly as the group responsible for the effect moves farther from the source, the strength of the acid is proportionately decreased.

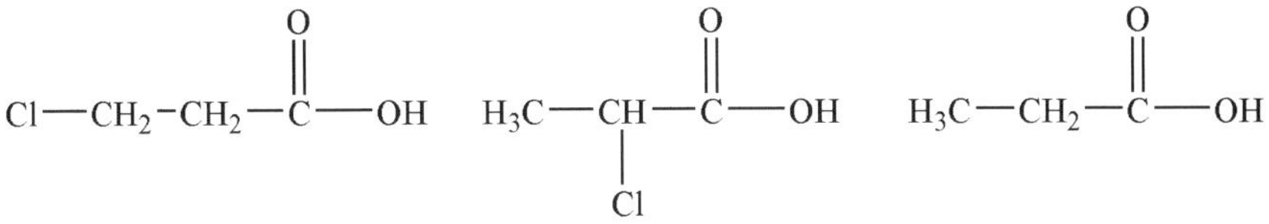

$$Cl-CH_2-CH_2-\overset{O}{\underset{\|}{C}}-OH \qquad H_3C-\underset{\underset{Cl}{|}}{CH}-\overset{O}{\underset{\|}{C}}-OH \qquad H_3C-CH_2-\overset{O}{\underset{\|}{C}}-OH$$

$$pK_a = 4.08 \qquad\qquad pK_a = 2.80 \qquad\qquad pK_a = 4.87$$

5) The presence of a group with +I effect decreases the acidic strength

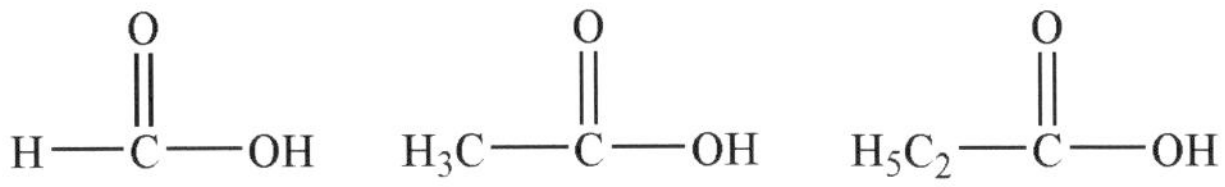

$$H-\overset{O}{\underset{\|}{C}}-OH \qquad H_3C-\overset{O}{\underset{\|}{C}}-OH \qquad H_5C_2-\overset{O}{\underset{\|}{C}}-OH$$

$$pK_a = 3.75 \qquad\qquad pK_a = 4.76 \qquad\qquad pK_a = 4.87$$

Acidity is primarily determined by the difference in stability between the acid and the anion. The main reason behind the release of the H⁺ proton by carboxylic acids is the existence of resonance structures for the acid and the anion:

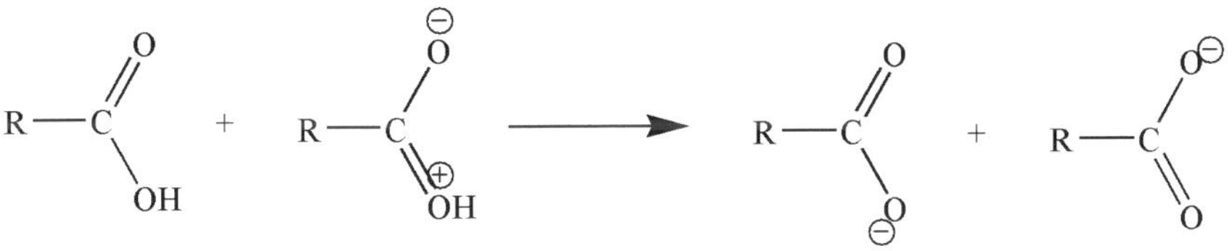

$$R-\overset{O}{\underset{\diagdown OH}{\diagup}} \quad + \quad R-\underset{\overset{\oplus}{OH}}{\overset{\ominus}{\overset{O}{\diagup}}}\diagdown \quad \longrightarrow \quad R-\overset{O}{\underset{\diagdown \underset{\ominus}{O}}{\diagup}} \quad + \quad R-\underset{\diagdown O}{\overset{\ominus O}{\diagup}}$$

$$\qquad\qquad \text{Not equivalent} \qquad\qquad\qquad\qquad \text{Equivalent}$$

Since resonance stabilization is so much greater for the anion than the carboxylic acid, equilibrium is shifted in the direction of increased ionization and thus the K_a is increased. The acidity of the carboxylic acid therefore exists because of this powerful resonance stabilization.

---> Quick Facts: *Basicity of Amines*

- According to the Bronsted – Lowry definition, a base is a substance that accepts a proton.
- Basicity is proportional to the base dissociation constant
- The basic character of amines is due to the presence of unshared pair of electrons on the N atom, which accept protons.
- The readiness with which the lone pair of electrons is available for co-ordination with a proton determines the relative basic strength of amines.

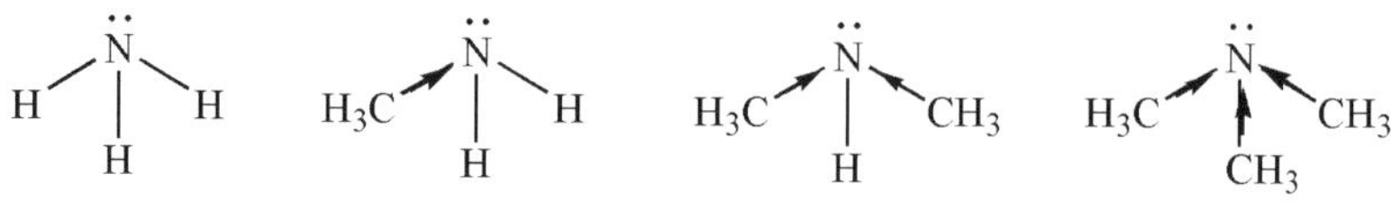

$$H-\overset{\cdot\cdot}{\underset{H}{N}}-H \qquad H_3C-\overset{\cdot\cdot}{\underset{H}{N}}-H \qquad H_3C-\overset{\cdot\cdot}{\underset{H}{N}}-CH_3 \qquad H_3C-\overset{\cdot\cdot}{\underset{CH_3}{N}}-CH_3$$

$$(1°)(2°)(3°)$$

- CH_3 group has a +I effect because it is an electron releasing group. As the number of Me groups increase, the lone pair of electrons on the N atom is more available to accept H^+. Therefore, on the basis of inductive effect, the relative basic strength order should be:

$$NH_3 < 1° < 2° < 3°$$

- But the basicity order is actually:

$$NH_3 < 3° < 1° < 2°$$

This anomalous behaviour of 3° amines is due to the presence of three bulky R groups which shield the lone pair of electrons on the N (steric effect) atom. Hence it is not readily available for protonation.

Chapter 2: Strength of Carboxylic Acids and Amines

Key Concept: Resonance Effect

The resonance effect implies the dispersion of electrical charges over several atomic centres caused by the movement of delocalized electrons. This effect makes the species more stable. For example, the following carbanion gets stabilized due to resonance effect.

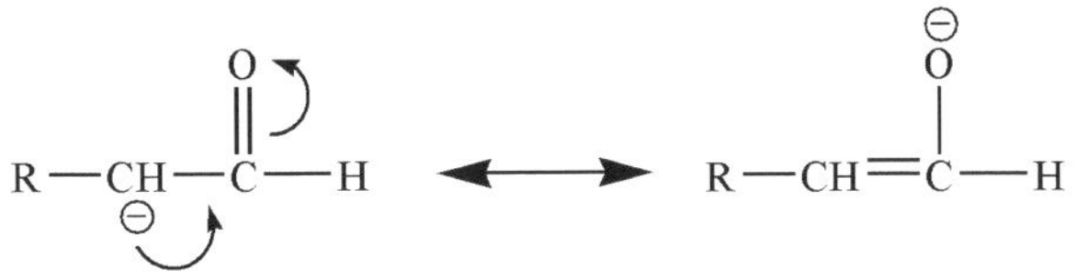

$$R-CH-\overset{O}{\underset{\ominus}{\overset{\|}{C}}}-H \longleftrightarrow R-CH=\overset{\overset{\ominus}{O}}{\underset{|}{C}}-H$$

A group that releases electrons to the benzene ring is an activating group. A group that withdraws electrons from benzene is a deactivating group.

Some of the general principles of the concept of resonance that are important to understand are as follows:

1) Whenever a molecule can be represented by two or more structures that differ only in the arrangement of electrons, resonance exists. This means that the molecule does not actually exist on one of these states alone, but is a hybrid of all of them.
2) When these structures are of approximately the same stability, then resonance is important.
3) The hybrid is more stable than any of the single contributing components

Certain criteria can be used to estimate the relative stability of resonance structures:

1) First, is if the structure seems reasonable, meaning that you may have come across a compound whose properties are accounted for by a structure of that type.
2) Electronegativity and location of charge.
3) Exceptions to the above rules in which overwhelming evidence indicates the existence of resonance structures.

Hyperconjugation is an extension of resonance theory in which a double bond is not involved. In this case, delocalization of the σ bond orbitals occurs. An example of this is shown below for the ethyl radical.

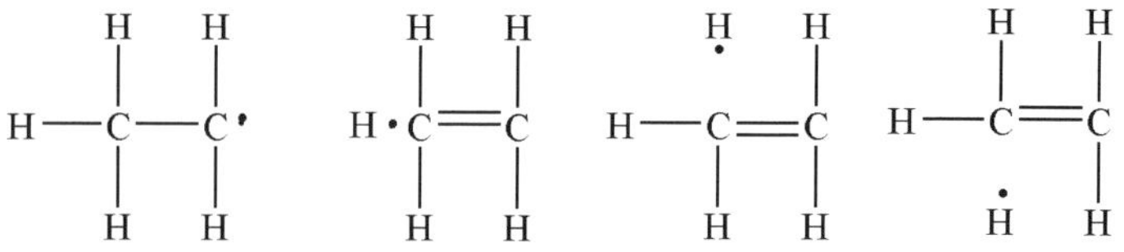

The ethyl radical is not simply structure I, but a hybrid of the additional structures as well. What this means is that the carbon-hydrogen bond is something less than a single bond with the odd electron partially accommodated by the hydrogens, and the carbon-carbon bond possesses some double bond characteristics.

GAMSAT Style Questions

Questions (1-5).

The pk_a is defined as $pk_a = -\log(k_a)$

1. Which of the following has the largest pK_a value?

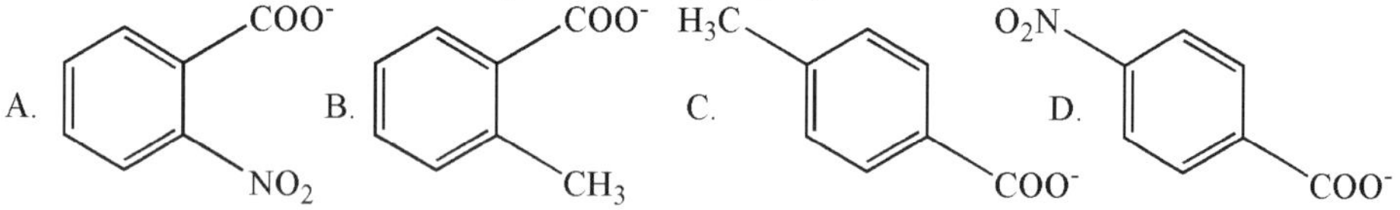

   A. benzene with COO⁻ and NO₂ substituents (ortho)
   B. benzene with COO⁻ and CH₃ substituents (ortho)
   C. benzene with H₃C and COO⁻ substituents (para)
   D. benzene with O₂N and COO⁻ substituents (para)

2. Which of the following order of increasing pKa value is correct?
   A. propanoic acid < α-chloropropanoic acid < β-chloropropanoic acid
   B. α - chloropropanoic acid < β-chloropropanoic acid < propanoic acid
   C. β-chloropropanoic acid < α - chloropropionic acid < propanoic acid
   D. β-chloropropanoic acid < propanoic acid < α - chloropropionic acid

Chapter 2: Strength of Carboxylic Acids and Amines

The greater the tendency to accept protons, the greater the basicity. The strength of the halogen substituted carboxylic acids decreases as the distance of halogen is increased from the carboxylic group.

3. Which of the following compound is the best proton acceptor?

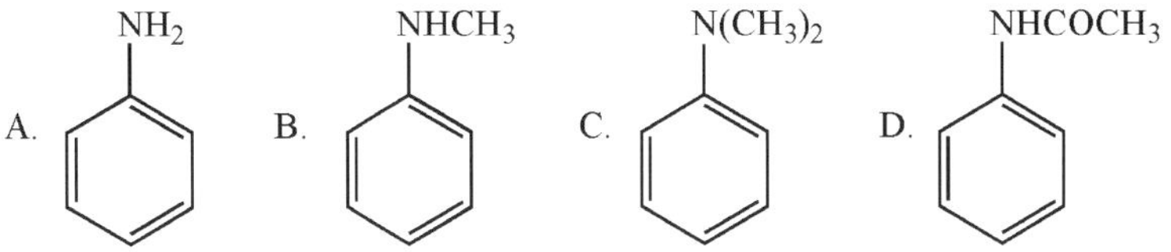

A. (phenyl)-NH$_2$ B. (phenyl)-NHCH$_3$ C. (phenyl)-N(CH$_3$)$_2$ D. (phenyl)-NHCOCH$_3$

4. Which of the following order is correct regarding the acidity of carboxylic acids?

A. CH$_3$CH$_2$CHClCOOH > CH$_3$CHClCH$_2$COOH > ClCH$_2$CH$_2$CH$_2$COOH
B. CH$_3$CH$_2$CHClCOOH < CH$_3$CHClCH$_2$COOH < ClCH$_2$CH$_2$CH$_2$COOH
C. CH$_3$CH$_2$CHClCOOH > CH$_3$CHClCH$_2$COOH < lCH$_2$CH$_2$CH$_2$COOH
D. CH$_3$CH$_2$CHClCOOH < CH$_3$CHClCH$_2$COOH > ClCH$_2$CH$_2$CH$_2$COOH

5. The acid dissociation constant is given by

$$RCOOH + H_2O \rightleftharpoons RCOO^- + H_3O^+$$

$$K_a = \frac{[RCOO^-][H_3O^+]}{[RCOOH]}$$

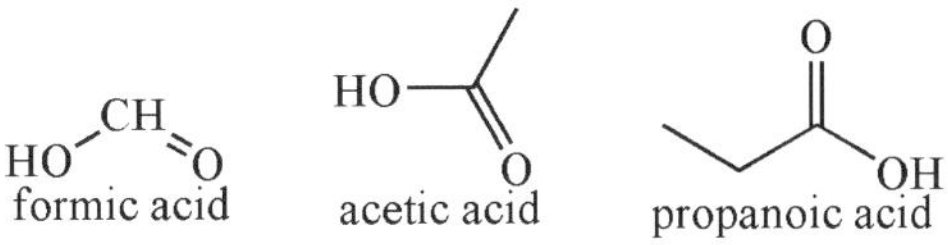

formic acid, acetic acid, propanoic acid

The correct order of decreasing dissociation constant is,
 A. formic acid > acetic acid > propanoic acid
 B. formic acid > acetic acid < propanoic acid
 C. formic acid < acetic acid > propanoic acid
 D. formic acid < acetic acid < propanoic acid

Question (6-10)

Carboxylic acids and their derivatives are some of the most important functional groups of organic chemistry. Carboxylic acids have a hydroxy group bonded to a carbonyl carbon; its acidity stems from the resonance stabilization of the deprotonated carboxylate ion, with the charge delocalized across both oxygen atoms. In carboxylic acid derivatives, the hydroxyl is replaced by another functional group. Esters have an alkoxy substituent, amides are bonded to an amine, anhydrides have another carboxylate group, and acid halides are bonded to a halogen.

Carboxylic acid derivatives can be interconverted through acid catalysis, when one substituent displaces another and the leaving group forms a condensation product with the acid proton lost by its replacement.

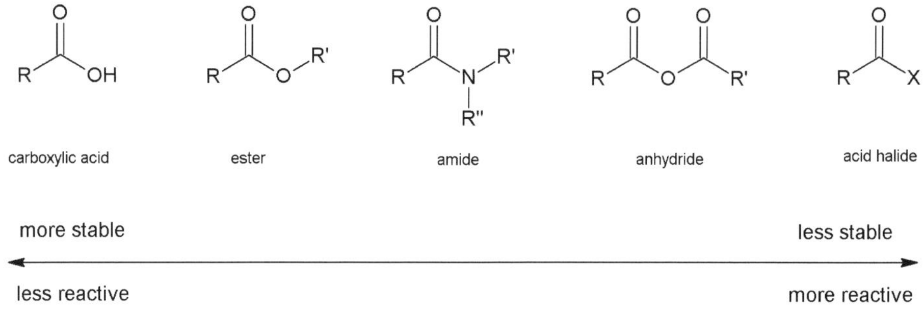

carboxylic acid — ester — amide — anhydride — acid halide

more stable ⟵⟶ less stable
less reactive ⟵⟶ more reactive

6. Which of the shown molecules is the missing reactant in the given carboxylic acid derivative conversion?

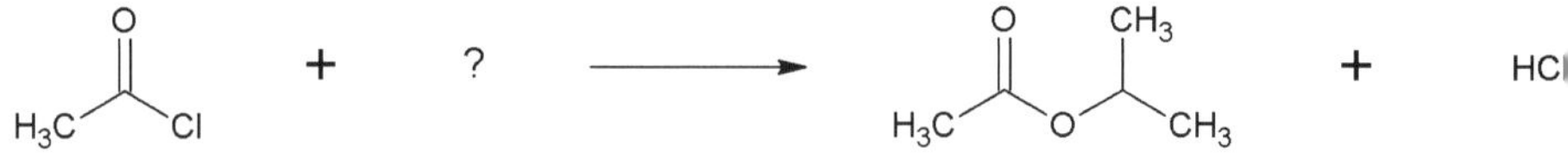

H_3C-CO-Cl + ? ⟶ H_3C-CO-O-C(CH₃)₂-CH₃ + HCl

A. H_3C-CH(CH₃)-CHO

B. H_3C-CH(CH₃)-CH₂-OH

C. H_3C-CO-CH₃

D. H_3C-CH(OH)-CH₃

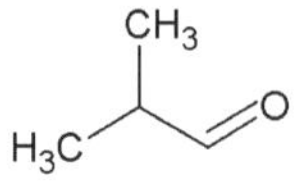

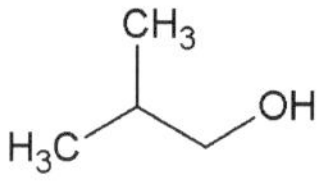

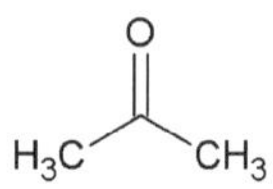

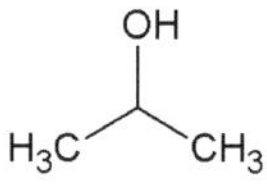

Chapter 2: Strength of Carboxylic Acids and Amines

7. What is the condensation product of the given carboxylic acid derivative conversion?

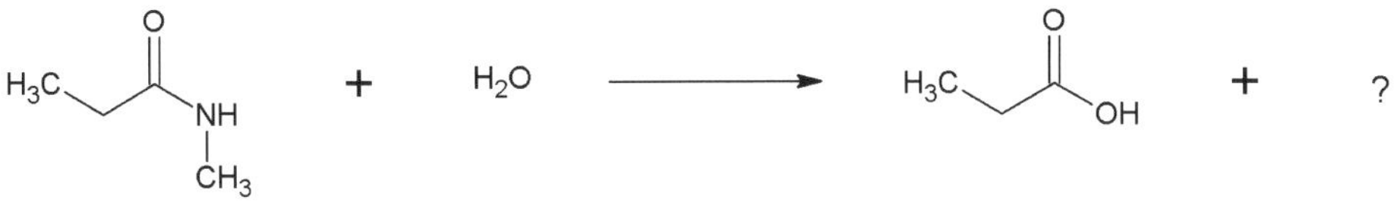

$$H_3C-C(=O)-NH-CH_3 \;+\; H_2O \longrightarrow H_3C-C(=O)-OH \;+\; ?$$

   A. ammonia
   B. a primary amine
   C. a secondary amine
   D. a tertiary amine

8. What will be the primary product when an acid halide is allowed to react with an aqueous solution of ammonia and an alcohol?

   A. a carboxylic acid
   B. an ester
   C. an amide
   D. an anhydride

9. Which of the following, when reacted with a carboxylic acid, will most favor the formation of an anhydride?

   A. an amide
   B. an acid halide
   C. an ester
   D. a carboxylic acid

10. Which of the following molecules can cyclize to form the products shown?

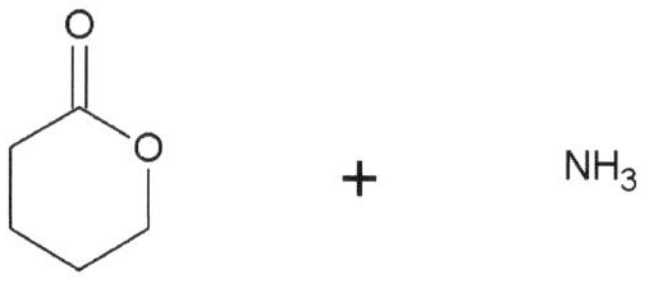

$$\text{(lactone)} + NH_3$$

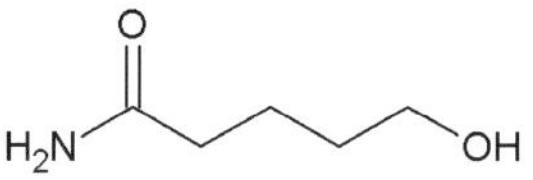

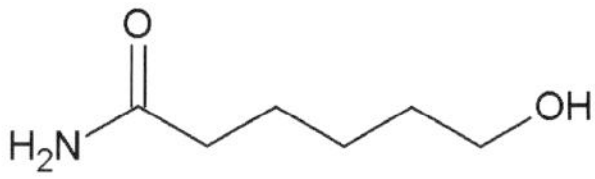

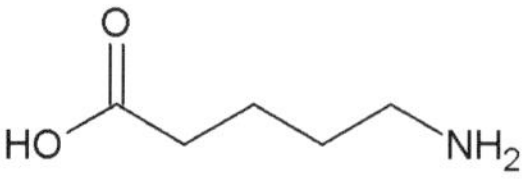

A. H₂N—(chain)—C(=O)—OH

B. H₂N—(chain)—C(=O)—OH (longer)

C. HO—C(=O)—(chain)—NH₂

D. HO—(chain)—C(=O)—OH

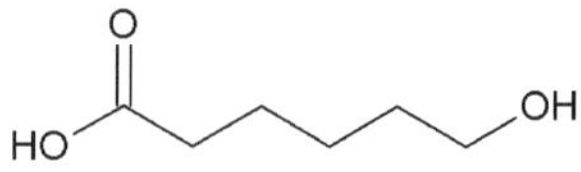

Question (11-15)

Amino acids are the basic building blocks of life, they form the proteins that are important to the development and function of organisms. Amino acids are characterized by a carboxylic acid with an amine bonded to the adjacent carbon, and varieties of side chains branching off the central structure.

Amino acids often have several different acidic or basic groups, leading to complex interactions within the molecule. Amino acids form proteins, or polypeptides, when the acid of one reacts with the amine of the next, losing water and forming a peptide bond.

11. How many tripeptides can be arranged using from the amino acids from the tripeptide shown?

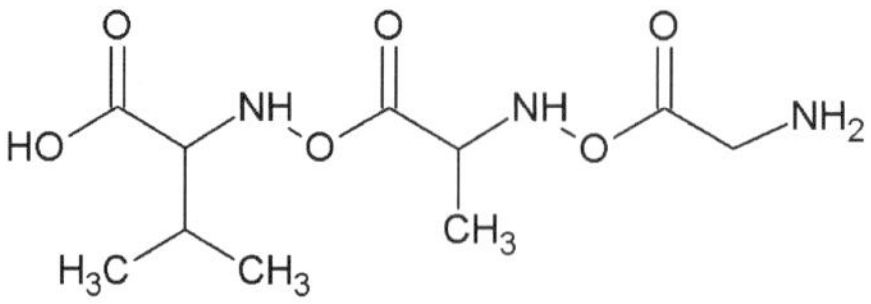

12. Which of the following is the correct order, from most acidic to least acidic, of the functional groups of the fully protonated form of the amino acid threonine?

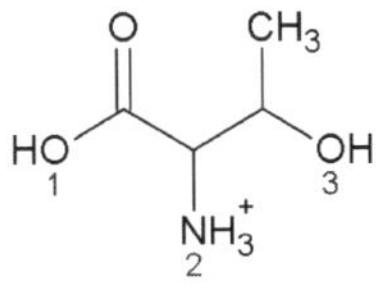

threonine

A. 1, 2, 3
B. 1, 3, 2
C. 2, 1, 3
D. 3, 2, 1

13. At which pH is glutamic acid (pKa1 = 2.19, pKa2 = 4.25, pKa3 = 9.37) most likely to have an overall neutral charge?

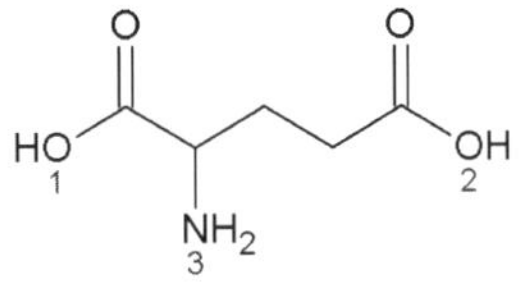

glutamic acid

A. 1
B. 3
C. 7
D. 10

14. Polypeptide bonds hold amino acids together in protein chains. What functional group is a polypeptide bond?

A. ester
B. anhydride
C. amide
D. azide

15. An electrolytic cell is created by applying an electric potential to a solution of the amino acid glycine (pKa1 = 2.4, pKa2 = 9.8)

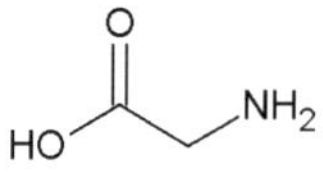

glycine

which is buffered to a pH of 11. The glycine moves toward the

A. cathode, because the amino acid has a net positive charge
B. anode, because the amino acid has a net positive charge
C. cathode, because the amino acid has a net negative charge
D. anode, because the amino acid has a net negative charge

Chapter 2: Strength of Carboxylic Acids and Amines

Solution

Question 1.

STEP 1 => What do you need to determine to solve the problem?
You need to determine which molecule has the largest pK_a value of the ones given.

STEP 2 => What relevant data provided in this problem is necessary in order to answer the question?
You are told that the pK_a = -log (Ka). This means that the larger the acid dissociation constant, the lower the pK_a and therefore, the more acidic the molecule.

STEP 3 => Use the relevant data to solve the question
The pk_a is defined as pk_a = -logk_a. The pk_a value and the acidic strength are inversely related. The weakest acid out of these four is C. Therefore, it will have the largest pk_a value. This is due to strong +I effect (electron releasing) of the methyl group at the p-position. Almost all ortho substituents increase the acidic strength of a benzoic acid. This is referred to as the ortho effect and is due to a combination of steric and electronic factors. Electronegative substituents such as N increase acidic strength because they cause destabilization of the benzene ring by electron withdrawal (-I effect). Therefore, the anion of the acid will be stabilized.

Question 2.

STEP 1 => What do you need to determine to solve the problem?
You need to determine the order of increasing pK_a value.

STEP 2 => What relevant data provided in this problem is necessary in order to answer the question?
You are told that the pK_a = -log (Ka). This means that the larger the acid dissociation constant, the lower the pK_a and therefore, the more acidic the molecule.

STEP 3 => Use the relevant data to solve the question
pk_a values are inversely proportional to the acidic strength. The presence of the electronegative Cl group results in electron withdrawal from the carboxyl group resulting in a destabilization of the acid and stabilization of the anion. This causes an increase in the strength of the acid. When the number of atoms between the electronegative group and the carboxyl group increase, the destabilization effect of the electronegative atom decreases resulting in a decrease in acidic strength. Therefore, the correct pk_a order is given is answer B.

Question 3.

STEP 1 => What do you need to determine to solve the problem?
You need to determine which molecule is the best proton acceptor.

STEP 2 => What relevant data provided in this problem is necessary in order to answer the question?
You are told that the more basic a molecule is, the greater its tendency to attract protons.

STEP 3 = > Use the relevant data to solve the question
The greater tendency of a molecule to accept proton, the more basic it will be. The most basic compound out of the four given is answer C. Due to crowding, there is a greater steric inhibition of resonance. The lone pair on the N atom is more readily available for protonation. Recall, actual basicity of amines is as follows: $NH_3 < 3° < 1° < 2°$.

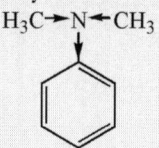

$$H_3C \rightarrow N \leftarrow CH_3$$

Question 4.
STEP 1 = > What do you need to determine to solve the problem?
You need to determine the correct order regarding the acidity of carboxylic acids listed.

STEP 2 = > What relevant data provided in this problem is necessary in order to answer the question?
You are told that the greater the distance of the halogen from the carbonyl group, the less acidic the molecule.

STEP 3 = > Use the relevant data to solve the question
Inductive effects are strongly dependent on the distance. The strength of the halogen substituted carboxylic acids decreases as the distance of halogen is increased from carboxylic group. The correct order of acidic strength is given in answer A.

Question 5.
STEP 1 = > What do you need to determine to solve the problem?
You need to determine the correct order of the dissociation constant.

STEP 2 = > What relevant data provided in this problem is necessary in order to answer the question?
You are provided with the equation for the acid dissociation constant. This tells you that the stronger the acid, the higher the value of K_a.

STEP 3 = > Use the relevant data to solve the question
The acid dissociation constant is given by

$$RCOOH + H_2O \rightleftharpoons RCOO^- + H_3O^+$$

$$K_a = \frac{[RCOO^-][H_3O^+]}{[RCOOH]}$$

As the size of R (alkyl group) increases, +I effect of R groups becomes stronger. The release of H from COOH group becomes more difficult. The acidic strength decreases. The acid dissociation constant decreases. The correct order of K_a is given in answer A.

Chapter 2: Strength of Carboxylic Acids and Amines

Question 6.
STEP 1 = > What do you need to determine to solve the problem?
The question requires you to identify the missing reactant in the conversion.
To do so you must identify what the structure of the product indicates about the reactants.

STEP 2 = > What relevant data provided in this problem is necessary in order to answer the question?
The passage indicates that the product is an ester, and that esters have alkoxy substituents on their carbonyls.
Since an alkoxide is simply a deprotonated alcohol (the proton catalyzed the conversion and bonded to the chloride), the reactant must be an alcohol with a structure identical to the right side of the product.

STEP 3 = > Use the relevant data to solve the question
Choices A and C are carbonyl compounds and therefore cannot be the reactant.
Choice B is an alcohol, but its structure is incorrect, as there is one more carbon than in the product. Choice D is an alcohol with the correct structure, and is therefore the reactant in the given reaction. The correct answer is D.

Question 7.
STEP 1 = > What do you need to determine to solve the problem?
The question requires you to identify the condensation product when the reactant shown is converted to the product.
To do so, you must identify the leaving group in the conversion.

STEP 2 = > What relevant data provided in this problem is necessary in order to answer the question?
The passage indicates that the reactant is an amide, and that an amine will be the condensation product in the conversion.
Also, the passage indicates that the condensation product will be the old substituent bonded to the catalytic hydrogen from the replacement substituent.

STEP 3 = > Use the relevant data to solve the question
Knowing that the condensation molecule is an amine does not narrow down the choices, but since the reactant shown has a single N-substituent, the condensation product must have a single carbon substituent as well.
This means that the condensation product must be a primary amine. The correct answer is B.

Question 8.
STEP 1 = > What do you need to determine to solve the problem?
The question requires you to identify the primary product of a reaction of several molecules.

To do so, you must identify which reaction is the most energetically favorable.

<u>STEP 2 = > What relevant data provided in this problem is necessary in order to answer the question?</u>
Therefore, it will readily convert to a lower-energy acid form. The passage indicates that the alcohol will form an ester, the ammonia will form an amide, and the water will form a carboxylic acid.

<u>STEP 3 = > Use the relevant data to solve the question</u>
All three of these are lower in energy than the acid halide, but carboxylic acid is the most stable and least reactive of all of the acid derivatives.
Also, water will be by far the most abundant reactant; therefore the majority of the acid chloride will react to form a carboxylic acid. The correct answer is A.

Question 9.
<u>STEP 1 = > What do you need to determine to solve the problem?</u>
The question requires that you identify the reactant that is most likely to form an anhydride.
To do so, you must identify which acid derivative is less preferential than anhydride.

<u>STEP 2 = > What relevant data provided in this problem is necessary in order to answer the question?</u>
The passage indicates that the acid halide is both the most reactive acid derivative and the only one less stable than anhydride.
Also, the carboxylic acid reactant is the necessary substituent to form the anhydride.

<u>STEP 3 = > Use the relevant data to solve the question</u>
Since the acid halide is the most reactive acid derivative, and since it is the only one that is less stable than anhydride, it must be the most favorable for synthesizing anhydride.
The correct answer is B.

Question 10.
<u>STEP 1 = > What do you need to determine to solve the problem?</u>
The question requires that you identify the reactant that forms the given product.
To do so, you must identify both the functional groups involved in the reaction and the carbon-chain structure of the reactant.

<u>STEP 2 = > What relevant data provided in this problem is necessary in order to answer the question?</u>
The passage indicates that an amine is the condensation product of an amide conversion. Also, the product is an ester, which is the product of an alcohol reactant. Finally, the diagram indicates that the product is a six-membered heterocyclic ring, including the ester oxygen.

<u>STEP 3 = > Use the relevant data to solve the question</u>

Chapter 2: Strength of Carboxylic Acids and Amines   49

Since the product must have an amide and an alcohol functional group, Choices C and D are not possible reactants.
Furthermore, the reactant must have exactly six atoms in the chain ending with the carboxyl carbon and the hydroxyl oxygen. Choice B has 7 atoms in that chain, and Choice A has 6. Therefore, Choice A has the correct functionality and structure and is the reactant.

Question 11.
STEP 1 = > What do you need to determine to solve the problem?
The question requires you to determine the number of tripeptides that can be arranged from the given molecules.

STEP 2 = > What relevant data provided in this problem is necessary in order to answer the question?
The passage indicates that amino acids can form peptide bonds to make proteins, or polypeptides.

STEP 3 = > Use the relevant data to solve the question
There are three different amino acids given, which can be placed into the first, second, and third positions in six different ways.
The asymmetrical nature of the peptide bond makes the direction of attachment a structural differentiation. Therefore, NH2-X-Y-Z-COOH is distinct from NH2-Z-Y-X-COOH, and six arrangements are possible (XYZ, XZY, YXZ, YZX, ZXY, and ZYX).

Question 12.
STEP 1 = > What do you need to determine to solve the problem?
The question requires you to order the functional groups from most to least acidic. To do so, you must understand the acid-base chemistry at work in the question.

STEP 2 = > What relevant data provided in this problem is necessary in order to answer the question?
The passage indicates that amino acids can have multiple functional groups with acidic or basic character, creating complex interactions.

STEP 3 = > Use the relevant data to solve the question
The carboxylic acid is the most acidic due to resonance stabilization.
The ammonium is the least acidic, as its amine conjugate base is fairly alkaline. The alcohol is in between, neither a good base nor a good acid. The correct order is therefore 1, 3, 2.

Question 13.
STEP 1 = > What do you need to determine to solve the problem?
The question requires you to identify the optimal pH for amino acid neutrality. To do so, you must understand the progressive acidity of amino acids.

STEP 2 = > What relevant data provided in this problem is necessary in order to answer

the question?
The passage indicates that amino acids can have multiple functional groups with acidic or basic character, creating complex interactions.

STEP 3 = > Use the relevant data to solve the question

Glutamic Acid

At pKa1 = 2.19 one of the carboxylic groups deprotonated and gave rise to a -1 charge on the carboxylate ion and +1 charge on the ammonium ion. i.e. net charge is zero. At half equivalence point only one carboxylic acid is deprotonated.
So pH = pKa = 2.19
This is close pH 3, so the answer is B.

Question 14.
STEP 1 = > What do you need to determine to solve the problem?
The question requires you to identify the peptide bond functional group.
To do so, you must understand what the peptide bond consists of.

STEP 2 = > What relevant data provided in this problem is necessary in order to answer the question?
The passage indicates that the peptide bond is the product of a carboxylic acid reacting with an amine, condensing water in the process.

STEP 3 = > Use the relevant data to solve the question
The condensation product of a carboxylic acid and an amine, in addition to the lost water, is an amide: a carbonyl carbon bonded to an amine, which is identical to a peptide bond. The answer is C.

Question 15.
STEP 1 = > What do you need to determine to solve the problem?
The question requires you to determine the effect of electrolysis on a buffered amino acid.
To do so, you must understand what electrolysis does.

STEP 2 = > What relevant data provided in this problem is necessary in order to answer the question?
The passage indicates that amino acids can have multiple functional groups with acidic or basic character, creating complex interactions.

STEP 3 = > Use the relevant data to solve the question
At a pH of 11, glycine will be fully deprotonated and have a charge of -1.
Since electrolysis involves applying electric potential to a solution, the negative glycine molecule will move towards the positive anode due to electric attraction. The answer is D.

CHAPTER 3: **Reaction Types: The GAMSAT Chemistry Challenge**

These types of questions occur quite frequently in the GAMSAT. This chapter has been prepared to familiarise you with the technique of solving these types of questions. You can gain a crucial edge over other candidates if you master the method to solve these types of questions as demonstrated in this chapter.

It is very rare that you will be asked directly on specific reaction types other than basic reactions such as acid/base, hydration, dehydration, addition, hydrogenation and esterification. You should already be quite knowledgeable on these basic reactions. More commonly, questions based on a passage will ask you to derive a product from a known reaction presented in a diagrammatical format. The general layout for such a question is as follows:

1) A passage explaining the reaction types and where they may be encountered.
2) A representation of the reaction in diagrammatical format showing the structural formulae of the reactants and the products.
3) Questions based on the passage and diagram where you could be asked several items.
    a. What is the product of the reaction for a given reactant?
    b. What is the reactant that produces a given product?
    c. Reasoning for a particular property based on the reaction.

The scope of reaction types that can be examined in the GAMSAT is very broad, they include the following:

- Reactions of aldehydes and ketones.
- Resonance stabilization reactions.
- Ketals and hemiacetals.
- Carbohydrates such as glucose, fructose.
- And they can utilize all forms of representation including Haworth and Fisher projections and structural formulae.

Listed below are some of the basic reaction mechanisms.

There are six basic types of reactions that occur
  A. Addition reactions such as halogenation, hydrohalogenation, and hydration
     1. Nucleophilic addition
     2. Electrophilic addition
     3. Radical Addition
  B. Elimination reactions such as dehydration
  C. Substitution reactions
     1. Nucleophilic aliphatic substitution with S_N1, S_N2 or S_Ni reaction mechanisms
     2. Nucleophilic aromatic substitution
     3. Nucleophilic acyl substitution
     4. Electrophilic substitution
     5. Electrophilic aromatic substitution
     6. Radical substitution
  D. Organic redox reactions
  E. Rearrangement reactions
     1. 1,2-rearrangements
     2. Pericyclic reactions
  F. Condensation reactions, where a small molecule (usually water) is split off when the two reactants combine

Here we will include a sample of the types of reactions that you may encounter, however, this is by no means a complete representation of the possible reactions that can be included in the GAMSAT and is only here to help further familiarize you with the topic.

Reaction of an acyl halide with water to form a carboxylic acid

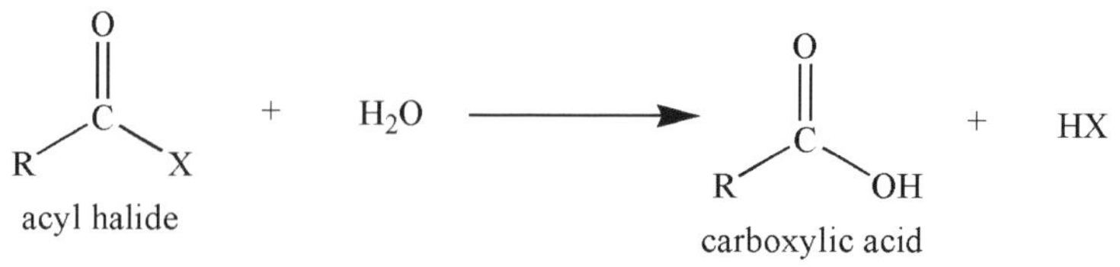

$$R-C(=O)-X \text{ (acyl halide)} + H_2O \longrightarrow R-C(=O)-OH \text{ (carboxylic acid)} + HX$$

Chapter 3: Reaction Types: The GAMSAT Chemistry Challenge

Halogenation of an alkene

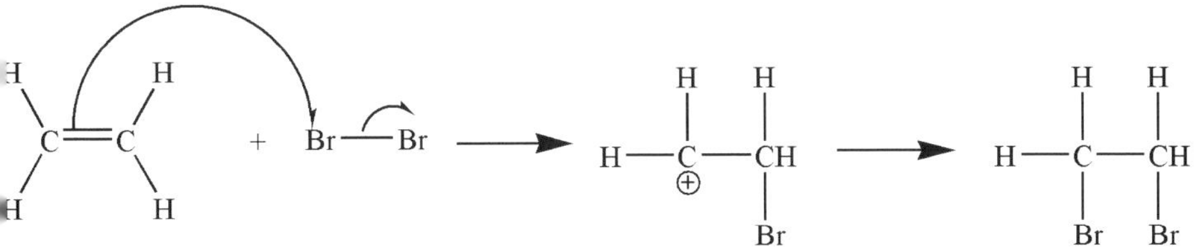

Formation of a secondary alcohol via reduction and hydration

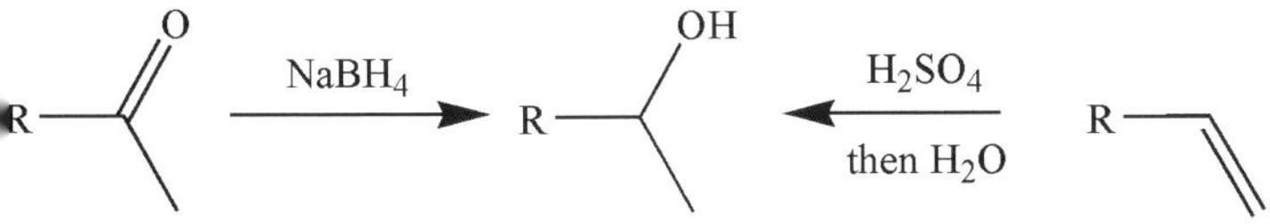

Hofmann rearrangement: Organic reaction of a primary amide to primary amine with one fewer carbon atom

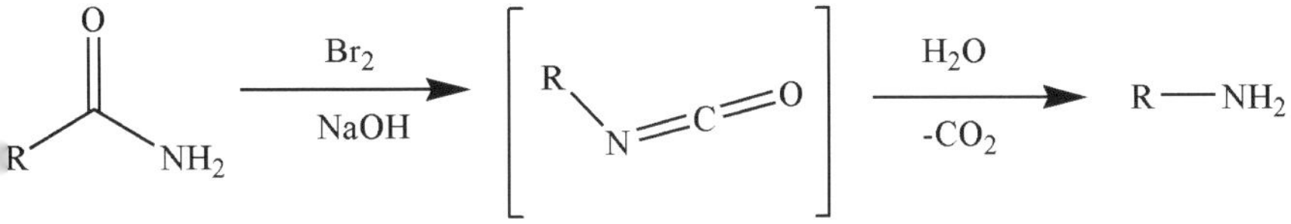

Friedel-Crafts reaction

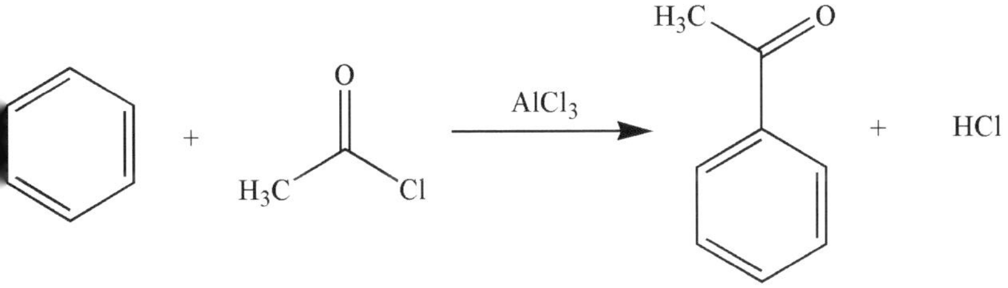

Lithium Aluminium Hydride reduction of a carboxylic acid to an alcohol

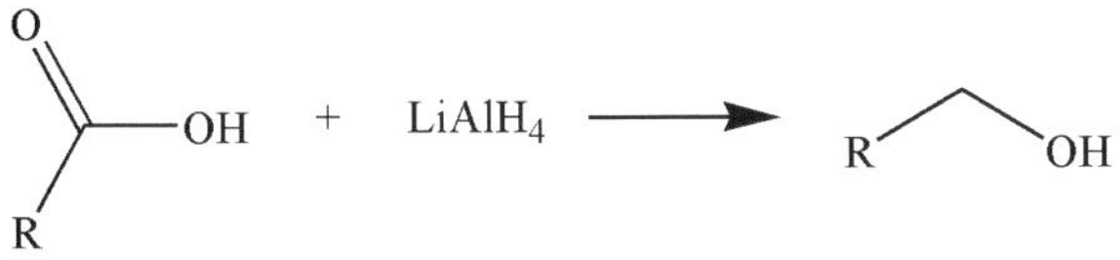

Cycloaddition

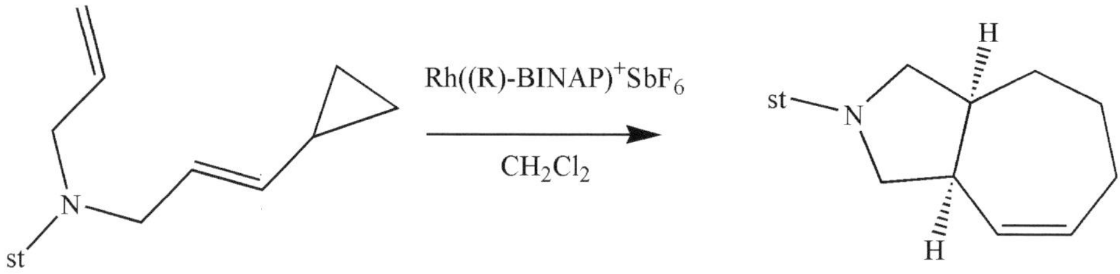

Favorskii rearrangement

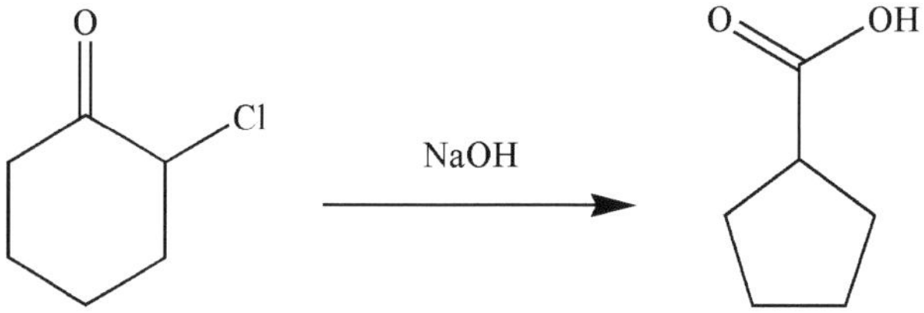

> **Tip:** For these questions, follow the PATTERNS! It is not necessary to know each and every reaction in an organic chemistry textbook. What is important is the process of thinking that allows you to arrive at the answer.

The only way to understand this topic is by working some example problems. Here we will list some of the basic reaction mechanisms.

Illustrative Questions

Question 1

1. The Aldol condensation reaction occurs when two molecules of either an aldehyde or a ketone combine. Under conditions of basic catalysis the α-carbon of one molecule becomes attached to the carbonyl carbon of the other. The product formed contains both an aldehyde and an alcohol functional group and hence is known as an aldol, making this type of reaction known as the aldol reaction.

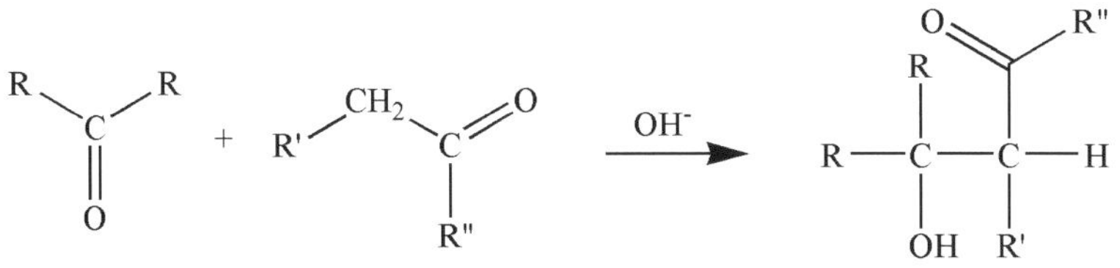

What structure represents the product of the aldol condensation reaction under basic conditions that occurs when 2 molecules of propionaldehyde (CH_3CH_2CHO) react?

A.

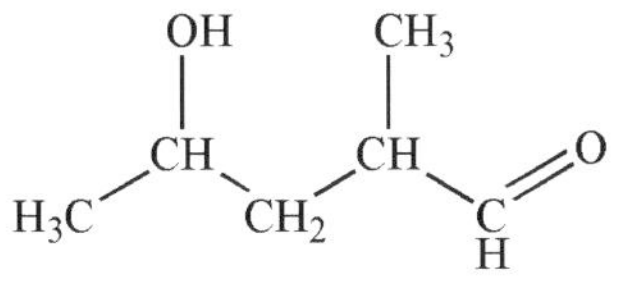

B.

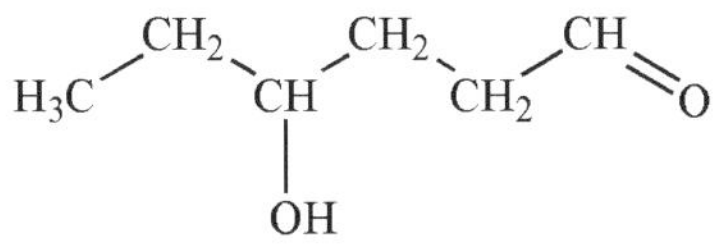

C.

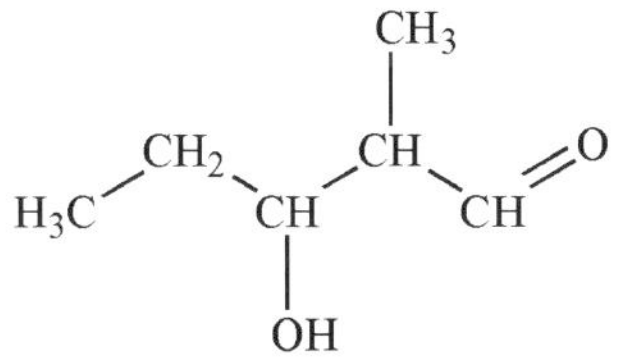

D.

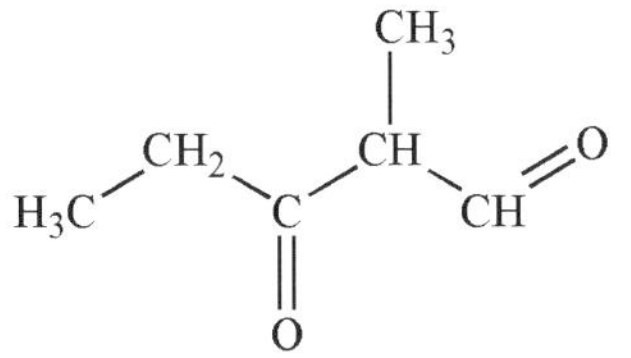

Solution

NOTE: In order to easily answer these questions, follow the three-step method described below.

<u>STEP 1 = ></u> What do you need to determine to solve the problem?
For this problem, we need to determine the product when two molecules of propionaldehyde react.

<u>STEP 2 = ></u> What relevant data provided in this problem is necessary in order to answer the question?
A general chemical reaction is given in the problem demonstrating the product of the reaction of two aldehydes or ketones under basic conditions. The reaction shown above demonstrates that when these two molecules react, the carbonyl carbon (the carbon double bonded to the oxygen molecule) of the first molecule represented will break one of the bonds with the oxygen molecule and bond with the carbon directly next to the carbonyl carbon of the second molecule. The oxygen that lost a bond will acquire a hydrogen thereby creating a molecule with both an alcohol (OH) group and a carbonyl (C=O) group.

<u>STEP 3 = ></u> Use this relevant data to solve the question
If you simply replace the R. R', and R" groups in the general reaction with the corresponding C's and H's in the reactants (propionaldehydes) from the question, you can then follow reaction in the question to obtain the answer. In this case, the carbonyl of the first molecule will break one of its bonds with the oxygen and form a new bond with the carbon directly next to the carbonyl carbon of the second molecule as shown:

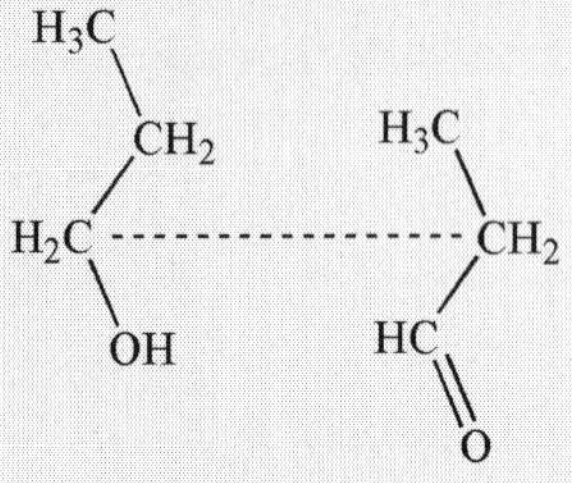

```
      H₃C
        \
         CH₂        H₃C
        /             \
   H₂C ---------------- CH₂
        \             /
         OH         HC
                      \\
                       O
```

So, examining the possible answers, you can see that C is the correct answer. A has the OH in the incorrect position, B has the incorrect C-C bond, and D has two carbonyl groups – the first carbonyl would need to be an OH group.

Chapter 3: Reaction Types: The GAMSAT Chemistry Challenge

AMSAT Style Questions

Questions (1-4).
Esters are usually formed by the reaction of alcohols or phenols with acids or acid derivatives. One type of reaction that an ester can undergo is alcoholysis (cleavage of an alcohol) of an ester. This process is called transesterification, which is demonstrated in the following reaction:

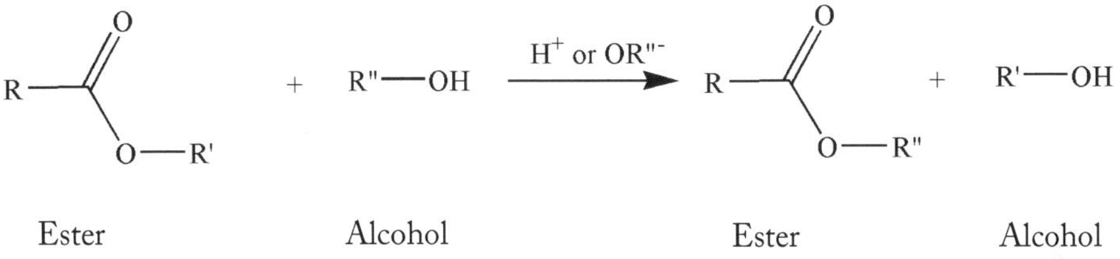

$$R-C(=O)-O-R' + R''-OH \xrightarrow{H^+ \text{ or } OR''^-} R-C(=O)-O-R'' + R'-OH$$

Ester   Alcohol   Ester   Alcohol

This reaction can be catalyzed by either an acid or a base and is an equilibrium reaction. The process of transesterification has been used to create Bio-Diesel fuel by taking a triglyceride molecule, or a complex fatty acid, neutralizing the free fatty acids, removing the glycerol, and creating an alcohol ester as shown:

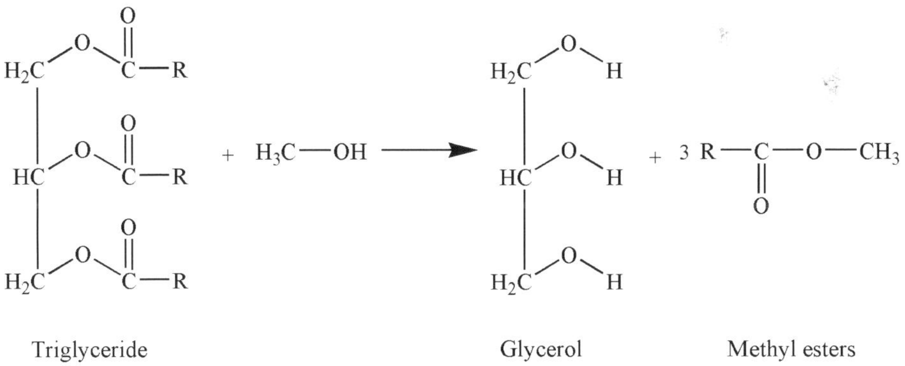

Triglyceride + H_3C-OH → Glycerol + 3 $R-C(=O)-O-CH_3$ (Methyl esters)

1. Which of the following two molecules will react in a transesterification process to produce the following products?

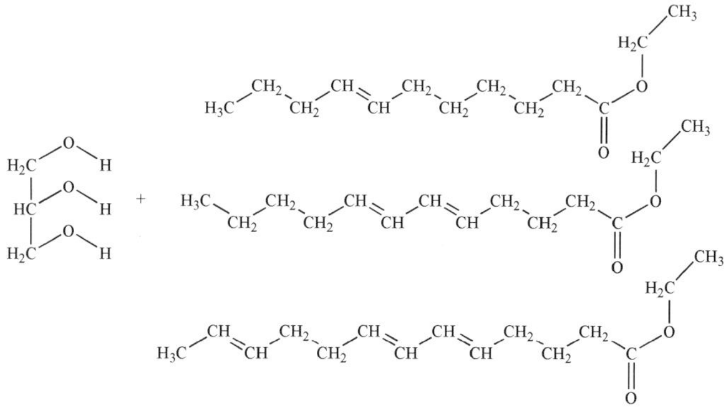

A. 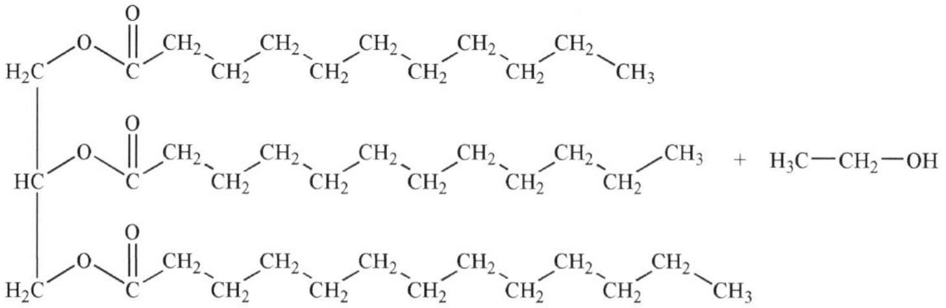

B. 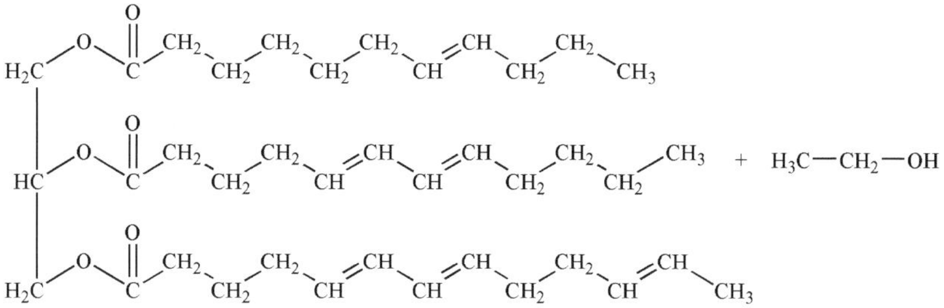

C. 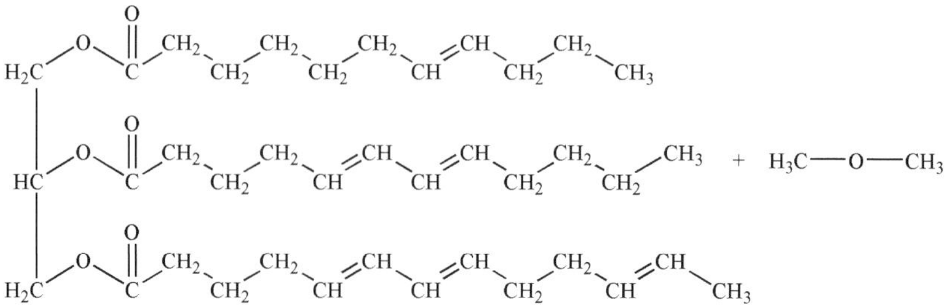

D. 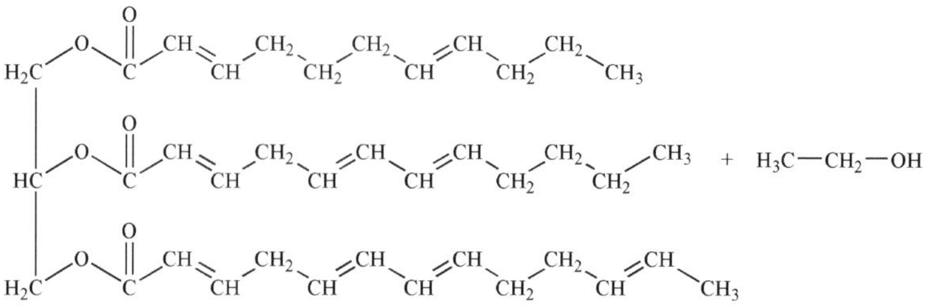

2. Consider the following structures
   I) $CH_3CH_2CH_2COOCH_2CH_3$

   II) $CH_3CH_2OCH_2COCH_2CH_3$

   III) 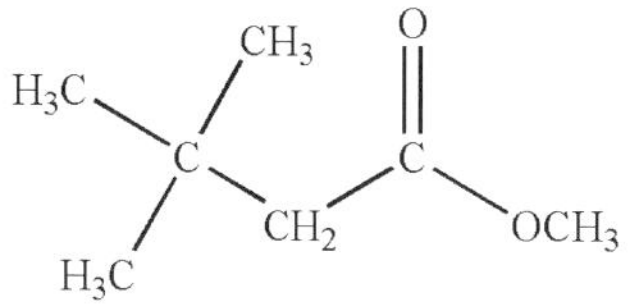

   (structure: a central carbon bonded to H$_3$C, H$_3$C, CH$_3$, and CH$_2$ which connects to C(=O)OCH$_3$)

   Which of the following would be able to undergo transesterification with methanol?
   A. I only
   B. II only
   C. III only
   D. I and III only

3. Which of the following molecules could be used to catalyze the transesterification process?
   A. HCl
   B. $CH_3CH_2O^-$
   C. H_2SO_4
   D. All of the above

4. Given the following reaction, what molecule corresponds to product P?

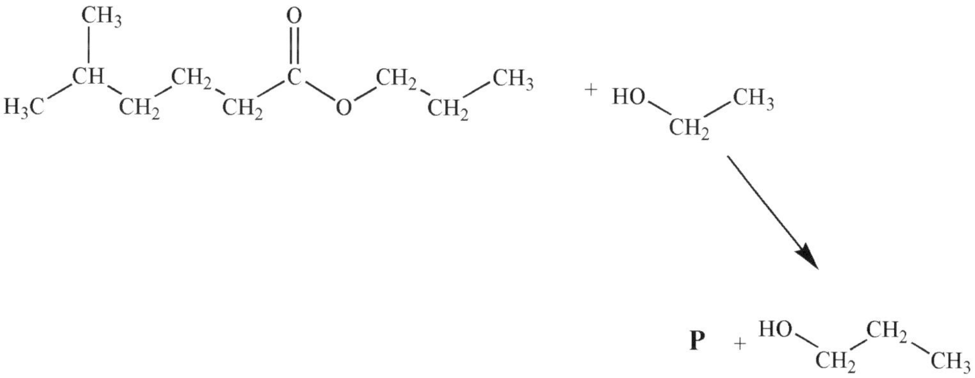

   H_3C—CH(CH_2CH_3)—CH_2—CH_2—C(=O)—O—CH_2—CH_3 + HO—CH_2—CH_3

   → P + HO—CH_2—CH_2—CH_3

A.

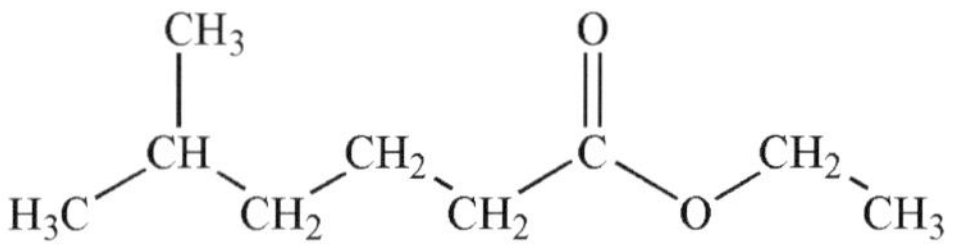

$CH_3-CH(CH_3)-CH_2-CH_2-C(=O)-O-CH_2-CH_3$

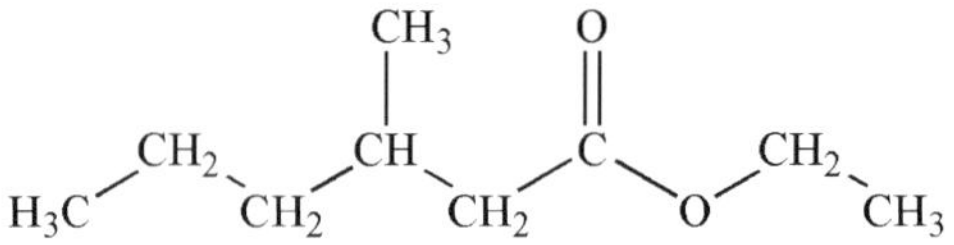

(structure A: H₃C–CH(CH₃)–CH₂–CH₂–C(=O)–O–CH₂–CH₃)

B.

(structure B: H₃C–CH₂–CH₂–CH(CH₃)–CH₂–C(=O)–O–CH₂–CH₃)

C.

(structure C: H₃C–CH(CH₃)–CH₂–O–C(=O)–CH₂–CH₃)

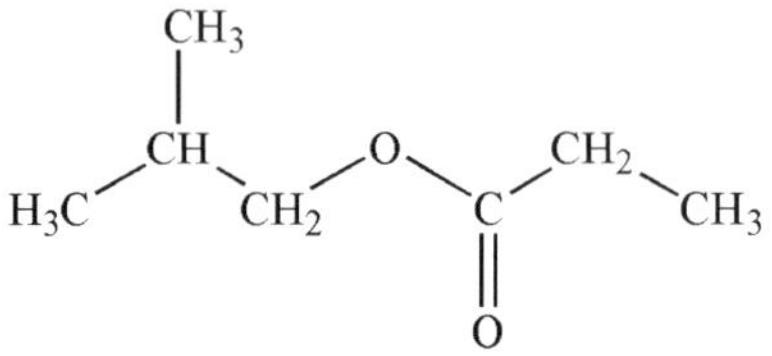

D.

(structure D: H₃C–CH₂–CH₂–CH₂–CH₂–C(=O)–O–CH₂–CH₃)

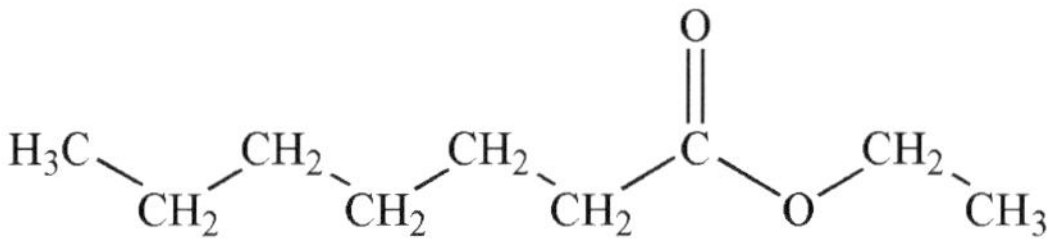

Questions (5-8).

Sigmatropic reactions are very important reactions seen in organic chemistry and involve the migration of a group with its σ bond within a π framework via a cyclic intermediate.

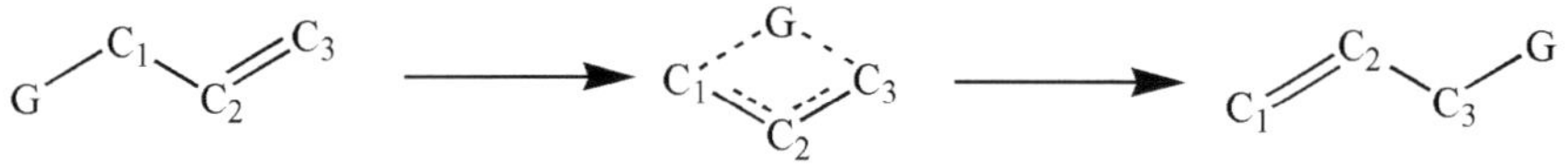

$G-C_1-C_2=C_3 \longrightarrow C_1\cdots C_2\cdots C_3 \text{ with } G \longrightarrow C_1=C_2-C_3-G$

In this simple example, the double bond between C_2 and C_3 breaks and forms a new bond between C_1 and C_2. At the same time, the G group breaks its bond with C_1 and forms a new bond with C_3 generating the resulting structure.

One example of a sigmatropic reaction occurs when aryl allyl ether is heated.

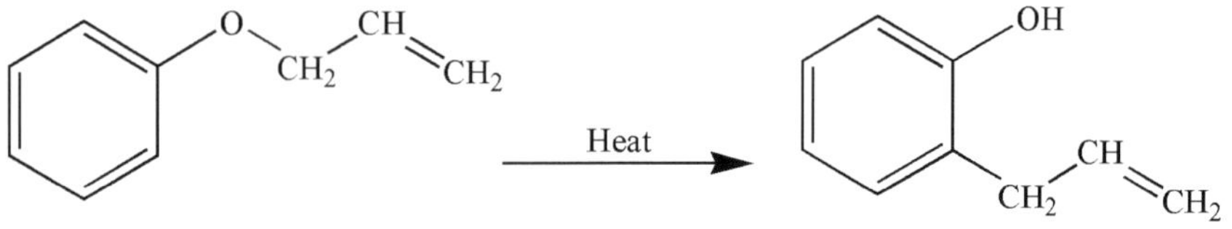

(Ph–O–CH₂–CH=CH₂) —Heat→ (ortho-allyl phenol: Ph(OH)–CH₂–CH=CH₂)

5. Using the above information, determine what the structure of the following molecule would be after undergoing such a reaction?

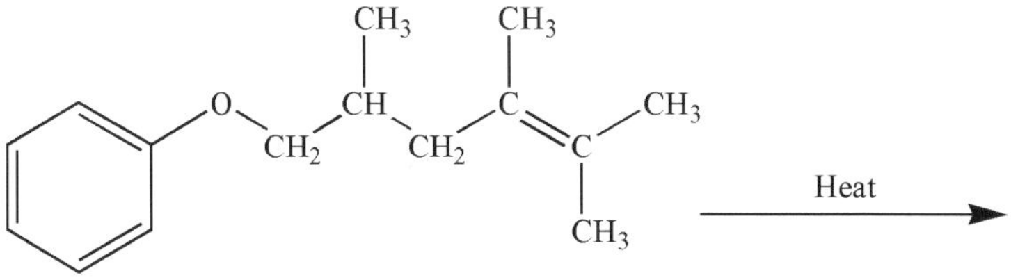

A.

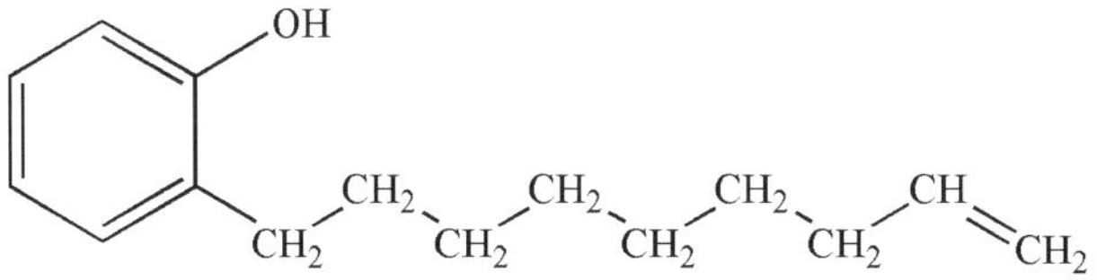

B.

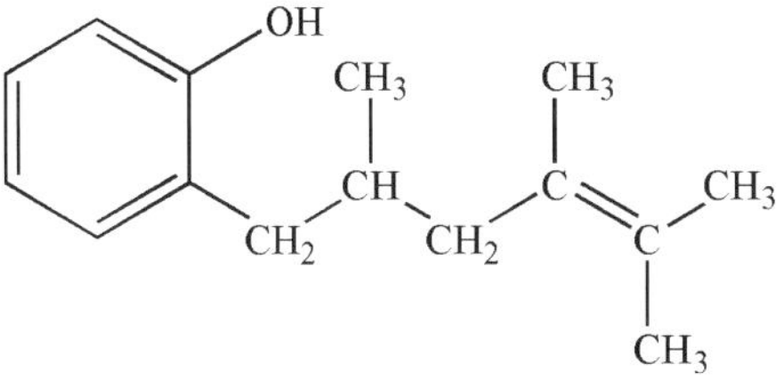

C.

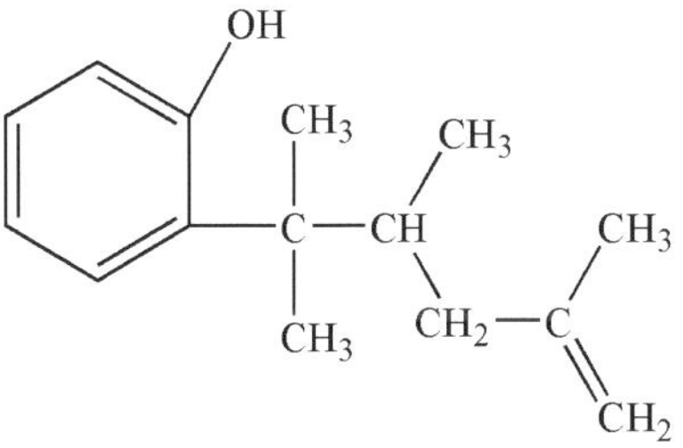

D.

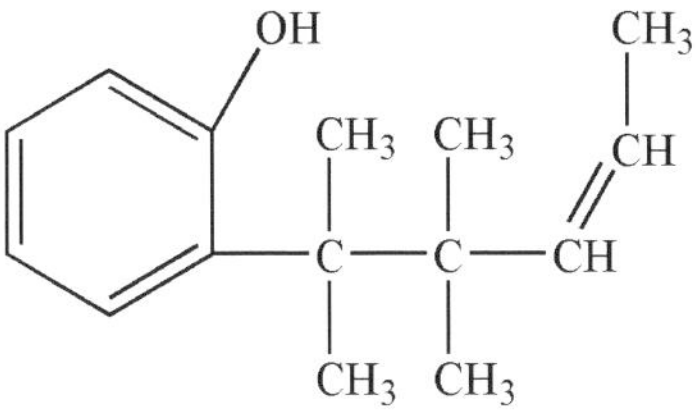

6. The following compound undergoes a thermal hydrogen shift when heated. Which structure could result from the sigmatropic rearrangement of the following molecule?

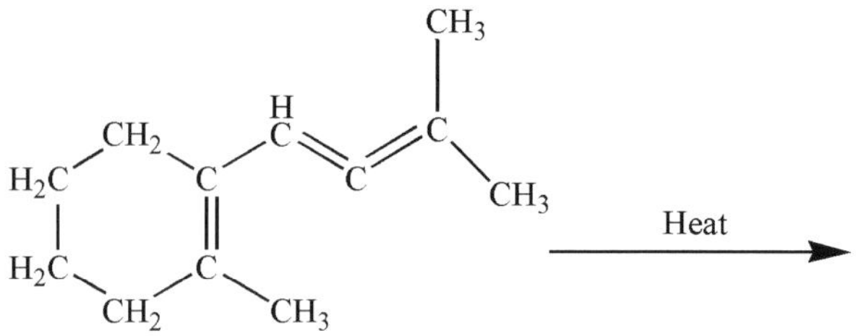

A.

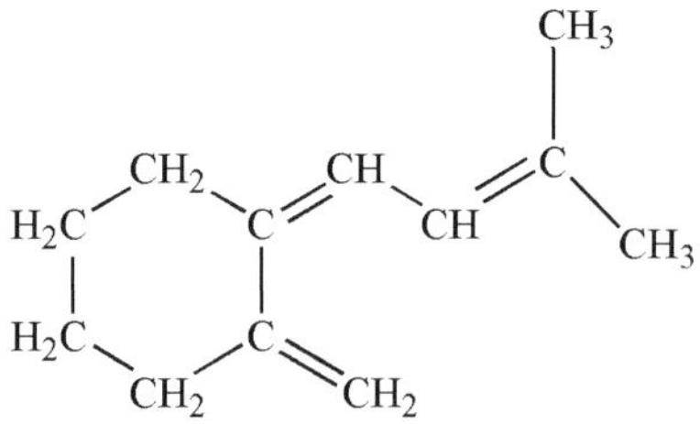

B.

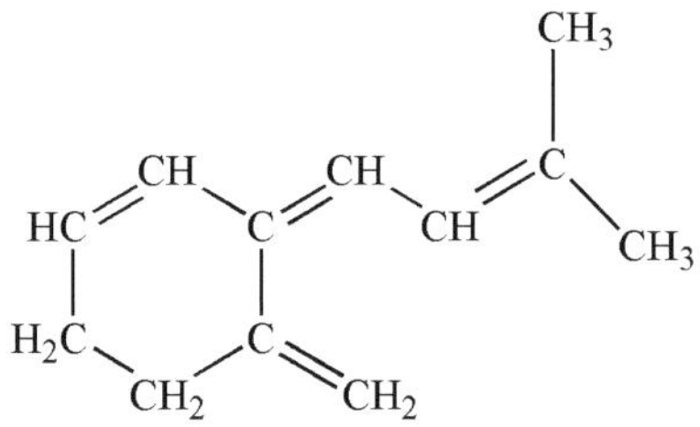

C.

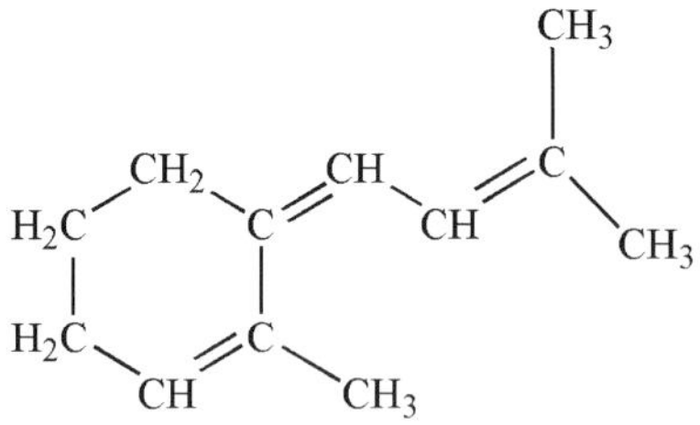

D.

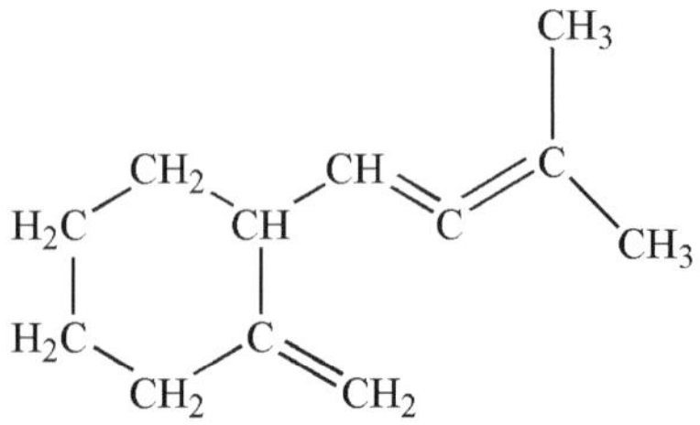

Many compounds that undergo sigmatropic rearrangements in nature may function as pheromones, antibiotics, and anti tumour agents. One such compound used by brown algae as a pheromone to attract male partners is shown below.

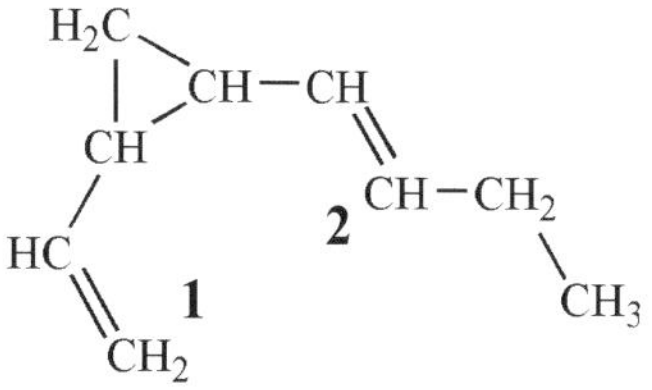

7. When this molecule undergoes sigmatropic rearrangement, a new bond will form between the two carbons indicated by the numbers 1 and 2 producing a carbon ring. How many carbons atoms will make up this new ring
   A. 6
   B. 7
   C. 8
   D. 9

8. How many double bonds will be in the new molecule formed?
   A. 1
   B. 2
   C. 3
   D. 4

Questions (9-13).

In the modern pharmaceutical industry, the aldol reaction is one of the most common reactions used in synthesizing complex drug molecules. The aldol reaction is very useful because it forms a new carbon-carbon bond, allowing chemists to create progressively larger molecules, and because it creates two new chiral carbons, allowing chemists to control the stereochemistry that is crucial for proper drug activity.

The aldol reaction consists of two sequential reactions that take place between two carbonyl compounds (aldehydes or ketones). In aldol addition, a carbon adjacent to a carbonyl group acts as the nucleophile, losing a hydrogen atom and attacking the electrophilic carbon of another carbonyl, reducing it to an alcohol. The aldol addition product can then undergo aldol condensation, in which the alcohol group and another hydrogen atom are eliminated, turning the newly formed carbon-carbon bond into a double bond. Generally, aldehydes are better electrophiles and ketones are better nucleophiles for the aldol reaction.

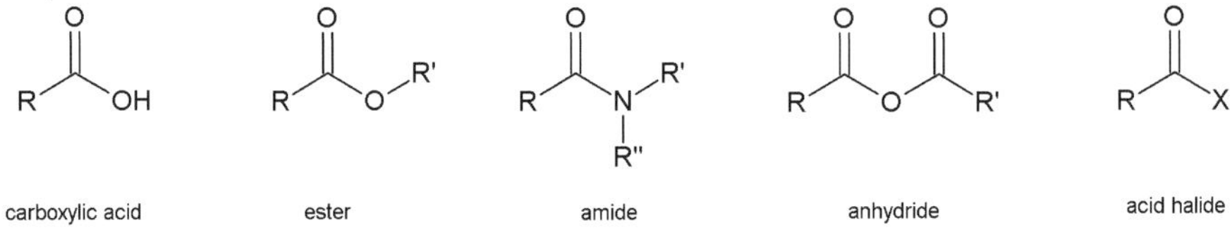

carboxylic acid	ester	amide	anhydride	acid halide

9. Which of the following is the product of the aldol condensation of Reactant A?

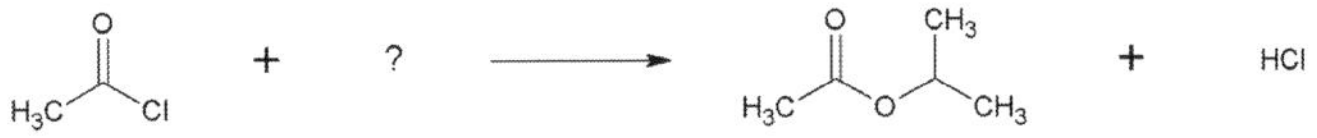

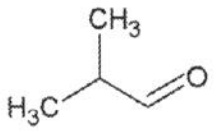

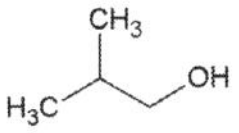

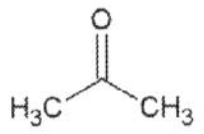

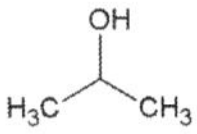

10. The aldol reaction of propanal and acetone yields a mixture of the following molecules. According to the passage, which of the following molecules is the major product?

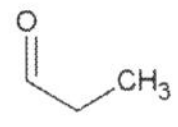

Chapter 3: Reaction Types: The GAMSAT Chemistry Challenge

propanal

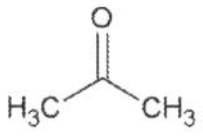

acetone

A

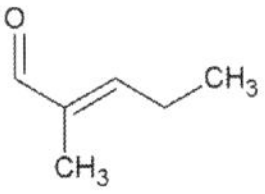

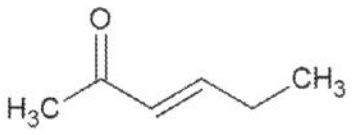

B

C

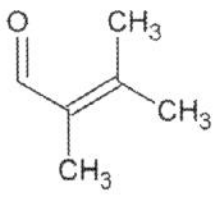

D

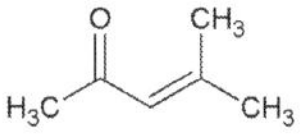

11. Which of the following reactants could form Product A in an aldol condensation?

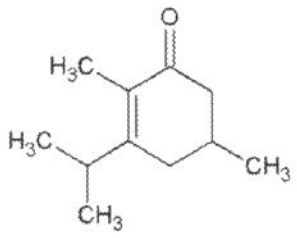

Product A

A

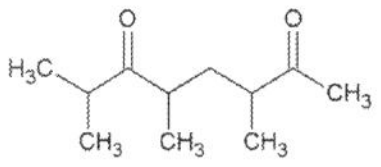

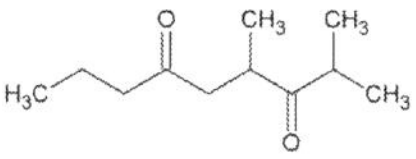

B

C

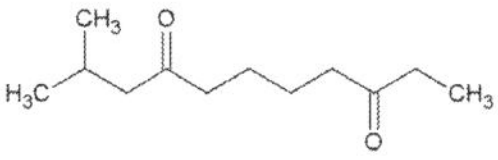

D

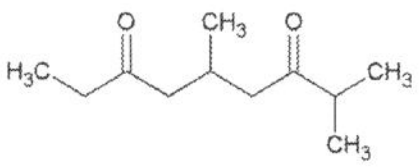

12. Which of the following reactants is capable of undergoing both aldol addition and condensation when reacted with itself?

A

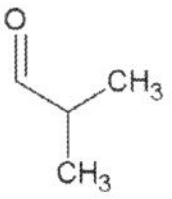

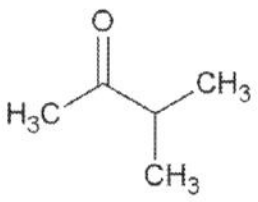

B

C

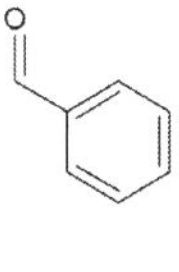

D

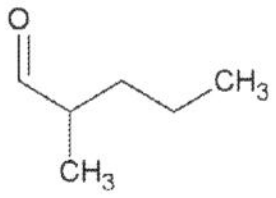

13. Which of the following molecules can be synthesized using an aldol reaction?

I

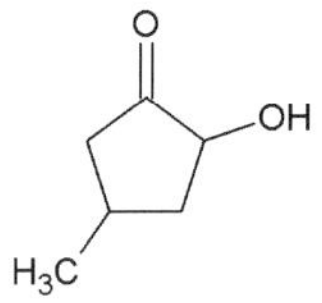

III

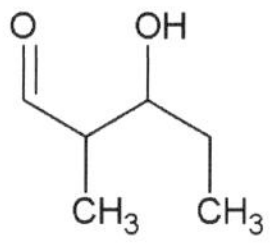

II

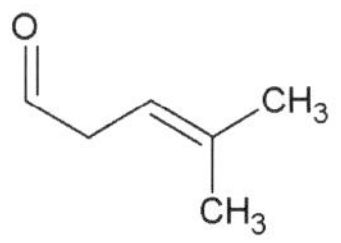

IV

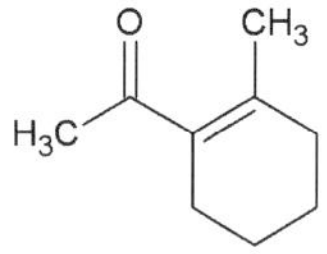

A. I and III only
B. III and IV only
C. II only
D. I, II, and IV only

Questions 14 - 18

A redox reaction is a chemical reaction in which the oxidation number of an element changes. The oxidation number describes the charge on an atom or species. Calculating oxidation numbers for relatively simple molecules is simply a matter of obeying a few basic rules.

First, any pure elemental atom or molecule, such as Ne or O2, has an oxidation number of zero. Next, the individual oxidation numbers of the atoms in any molecule or ion must add to the total charge on it. For example, the Na+ ion has a charge of +1, so the oxidation number of sodium is 1, and the oxidation numbers of the nitrate ion (NO3-) must add up to -1. Finally, within multiatomic species, oxygen typically has an oxidation number of -2; other oxidation numbers can be calculated to arrive at the charge on the species.

In a redox reaction, one or more elements lose electrons, making their oxidation numbers more positive (oxidation), while others gain electrons, making their oxidation numbers more negative (reduction). The species which loses electrons in the transfer, enabling another species to be reduced, is the reducing agent, while the species which gains electrons is the oxidizing agent.

Chapter 3: Reaction Types: The GAMSAT Chemistry Challenge

14. In which of the following molecules is the oxidation number of chlorine +5?
    A. NaCl
    B. $NaClO_2$
    C. $NaClO_3$
    D. $NaClO_4$

15. In the redox reaction

    $CuSO_4 + AgCl \rightarrow CuCl + AgSO_4$

    which element is reduced?
    A. Cu
    B. S
    C. Ag
    D. Cl

16. In the reaction from the previous question, which species is the reducing agent?

    A. $CuSO_4$
    B. AgCl
    C. AgCl
    D. $ZnSO_4$

17. Which of the following unbalanced reactions is a redox reaction?

    A. $CaO + KCl \rightarrow CaCl_2 + K_2O$
    B. $HCl + NaOH \rightarrow NaCl + H_2O$
    C. $AlPO_4 + MgSO_4 \rightarrow Al_2(SO_4)_3 + Mg_3(PO4)_2$
    D. $TiBr_2 + CoBr_3 \rightarrow TiBr_3 + CoBr_2$

18. In the following reaction, how many moles of electrons are transferred per mole of metallic iron reacted?

    $PbO_2 + Fe\ (s) \rightarrow PbO + FeO$

    A. 1
    B. 2
    C. 3
    D. 4

Questions 19 - 23

Aromatic compounds are unsaturated cyclic compounds, so named for their distinct odor, and important for their highly stable nature. The stability of aromatic compounds is derived from the interactions of π-electrons in the overlapping p-orbitals of the planar ring. An aromatic compound is a planar ring or rings overlapping p-orbitals projecting vertically above and below the ring plane. These p-orbitals can be involved in double bonding, contain an unbonded pair of electrons like in nitrogen or a carbanion, or be empty, such as in a carbocation. Aromaticity is dependent on the number of electrons located in this π-overlap bond: if the number of electrons can be represented as 4n+2 (2, 6, 10, etc.), the molecule is aromatic and highly stable. If the number of electrons is 4n (4, 8, 12, etc.), the molecule is antiaromatic and is highly destabilized.

19. Which of the following cyclic ions are antiaromatic?

I — cyclopropenyl with CH⁻
II — cyclopropenyl with CH⁺
III — cyclopentadienyl with CH⁻
IV — cyclopentadienyl with CH⁺

20. Of the heterocyclic aromatic molecules A and B, which nitrogen one pair is more reactive?

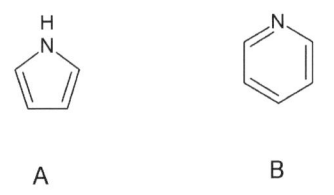

A — pyrrole (N-H)
B — pyridine

A. A, because its lone pair contributes to aromaticity
B. A, because its lone pair does not contribute to aromaticity
C. B, because its lone pair contributes to aromaticity
D. B, because its lone pair does not contribute to aromaticity

21. Which of the following molecules is the least stable?

A 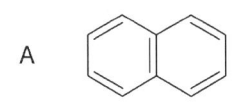   B

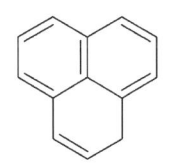

C   D

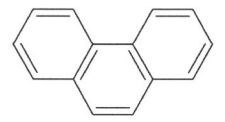

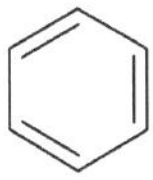

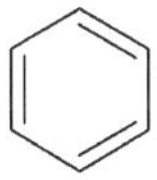

22. Which of the following molecules are aromatic?

I   II

III 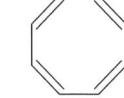   IV

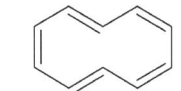

A. I only
B. II and IV only
C. I and III only
D. II, III, and IV only

23. What bond angle results in the least stress in an aromatic ring?

A. 90°
B. 109°
C. 120°
D. 135°

Question 24 to 28

The Diels-Alder reaction is a cyclization reaction that forms an unsaturated six-membered ring. The Diels-Alder reaction takes place between a diene and a dienophile. The diene can be any unsaturated molecule with two double bonds separated by a single bond; the dienophile can be any double or triple bond. The dienophile lines up each end of its bond to one of the double bonds of the diene. The π-electron system of the diene reacts with that of the dienophile, forming two new bonds from the far carbon of both double bonds to the dienophile and using the remaining pair of electrons to form a new double bond at the bond between the two original double bonds.

If the dienophile is a triple bond, then it becomes a double bond after the Diels-Alder reaction. Also, the Diels-Alder reaction can proceed with almost any substituents on the diene and dienophile; however, the mechanism of the π-interaction favors 1,2- and 1,4-substituted products over 1,3-substituted products when possible.

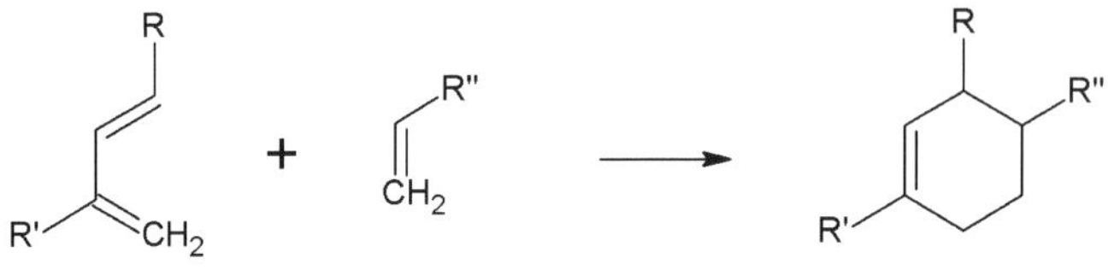

24. Which of the following molecules is a product of the Diels-Alder reaction shown?

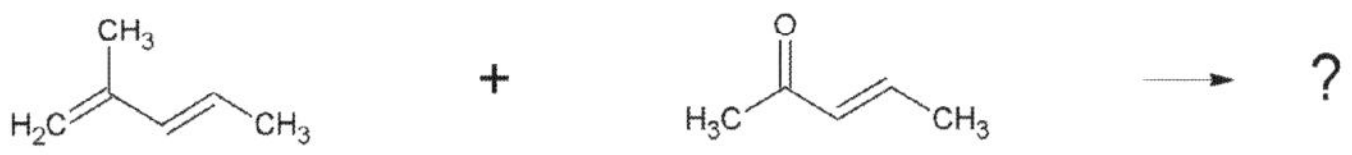

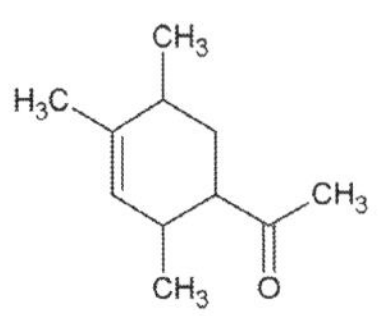

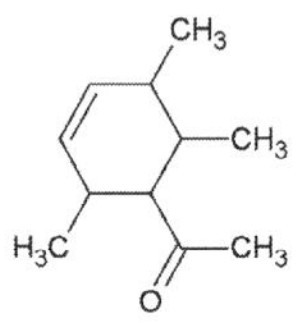

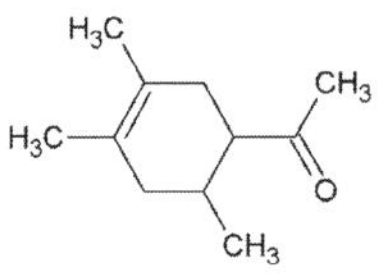

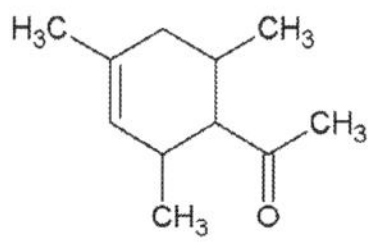

25. Which of the molecules below is the product of a Diels-Alder reaction involving a Diels-Alder product?

A 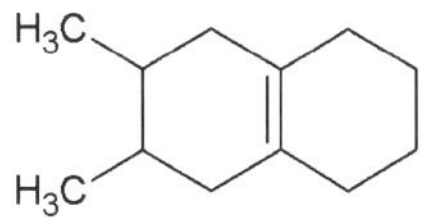 B 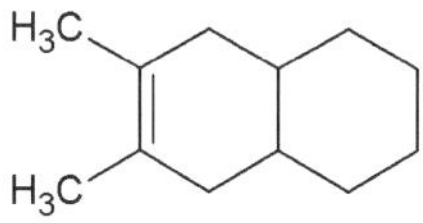 C 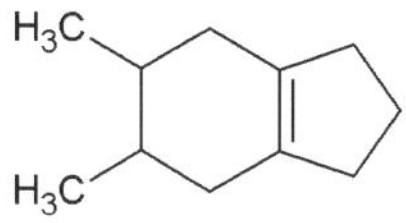 D

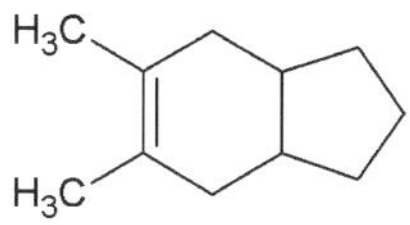

26. Which of the following pairs of reactants could form the Diels-Alder Product A?

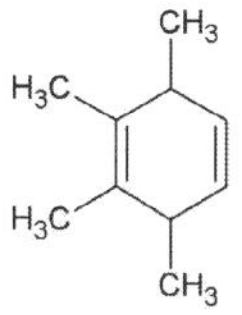

I

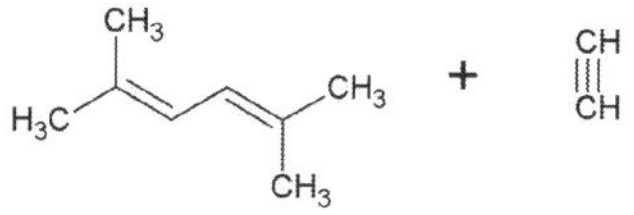

II

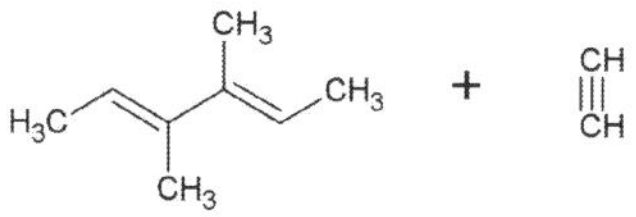

III

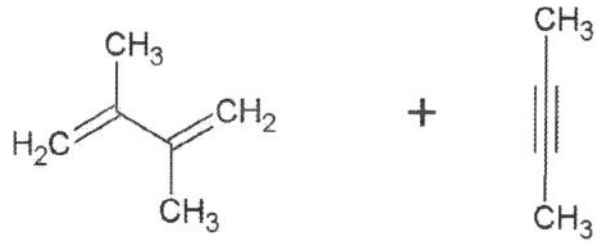

IV

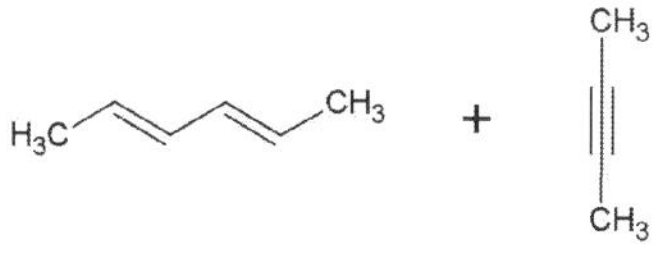

A. I only
B. II and III only
C. II and IV only
D. I, III, and IV only

27. How many different Diels-Alder products can be formed by the reaction of Compound A with itself?

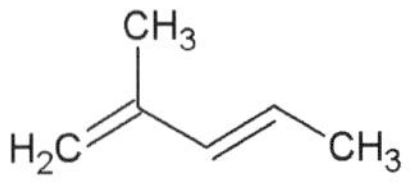

Compound A

28. Which of the compounds below is the major product of the given Diels-Alder reaction?

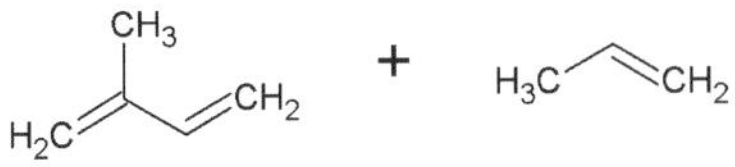

A

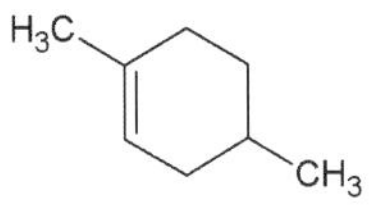

B

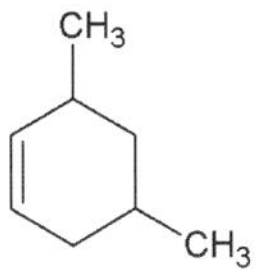

C

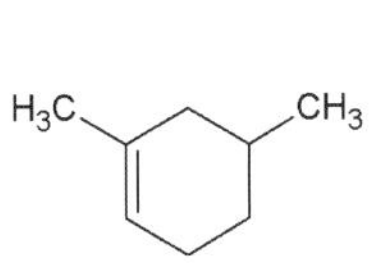

D

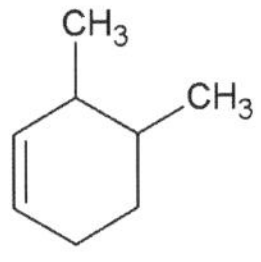

Question 29 to 33

Substitution is one of the most basic reactions of organic chemistry. In a typical substitution reaction, a substituent on an alkyl chain, often a halide, serves as a leaving group while a nucleophile takes its place. The nucleophile can be any species with free electrons that will bond to the carbon atom, which is partially positive due to the electron-withdrawing properties of the leaving group. There are two main mechanisms by which substitution reactions proceed, S_N1 and S_N2.

S_N1 reactions, or first-order substitution reactions, is so named because the rate of the reaction depends only on one molecule. S_N1 reactions are most common when the leaving group is sterically obstructed by bulky carbon-chain structure and the nucleophile cannot position itself to attack the carbon directly. S_N1 reactions proceed through a carbocation intermediate, which is stabilized by the high alkyl substitution on the carbon, and therefore the product of a chiral reactant is not stereospecific and is a racemic mixture.

S_N2 reactions, or second-order substitutions, are so named because the rate is dependent on both the alkyl halide and the nucleophile. The nucleophile positions itself to attack from directly opposite the leaving group, and the intermediate is a pentacoordinate structure. This arrangement leads to the inversion of stereochemistry in a chiral substitution.

29. Which of the following molecules is the S_N2 substitution product of the reactants shown?

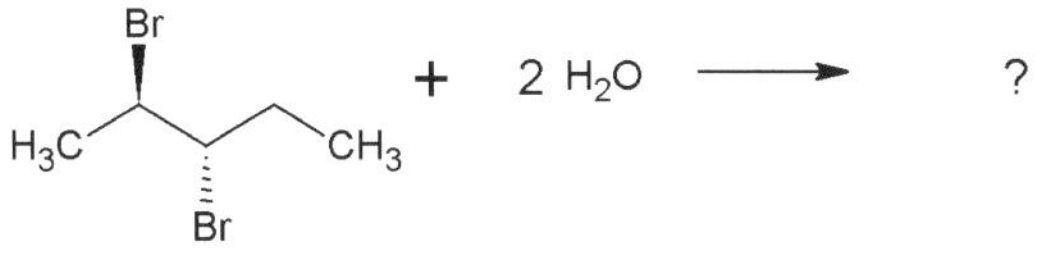

[Reactant structure: 2,3-dibromobutane] + 2 H₂O → ?

A. [structure with OH (wedge up), CH₃, OH (dash down)] H₃C-CH(OH)-CH(OH)-CH₃

B. [structure with OH (wedge up), OH (wedge up)] H₃C-CH(OH)-CH(OH)-CH₃

C. [structure with OH (dash), OH (dash)] H₃C-CH(OH)-CH(OH)-CH₃

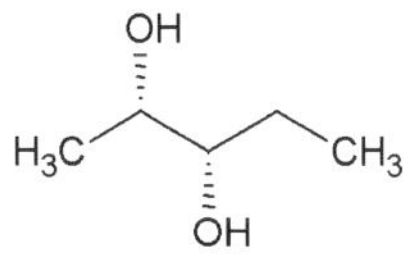

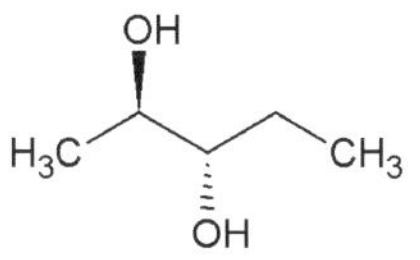

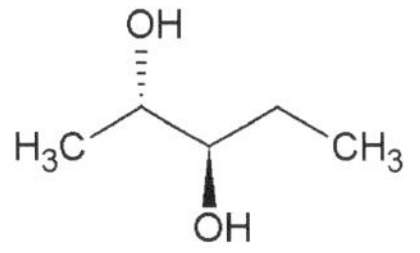

D. [structure with OH (up), OH (down)] H₃C-CH(OH)-CH(OH)-CH₃

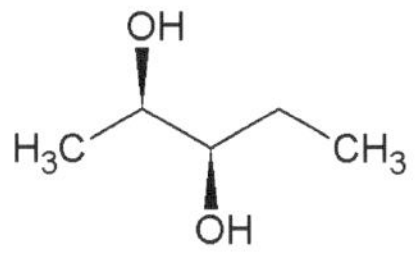

30. Which substitution mechanism will this reaction most likely follow?

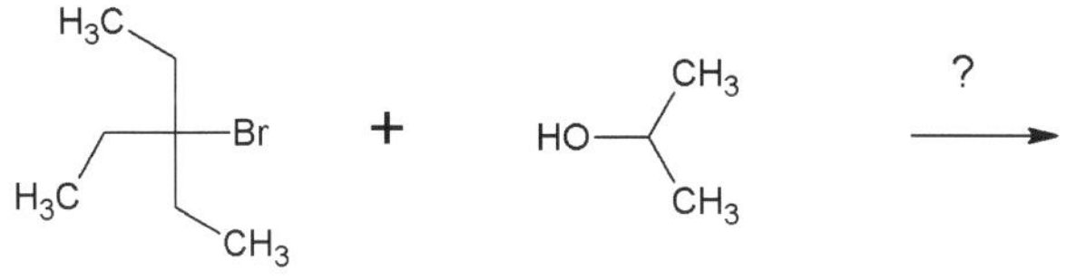

[(CH₃)₃C-Br] + HO-CH(CH₃)₂ → ?

A. S_N2, because the nucleophile is not a bulky base.
B. S_N2, because the alkyl halide is not sterically hindered.
C. S_N1, because the nucleophile is a weak base.
D. S_N1, because the alkyl halide is sterically hindered.

31. Which mechanism did the substitution reaction that resulted in this product most likely follow?

95% 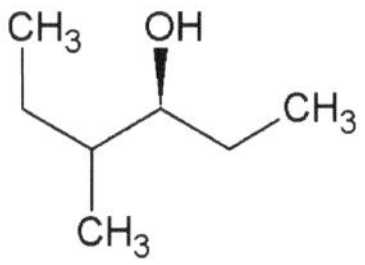

A. S_N2, because the primary product is stereospecific at the site of substitution.
B. S_N2, because the hydroxide ion is a strong base.
C. S_N1, because a secondary alkyl halide is sterically hindered.
D. S_N1, because only one of the chiral carbons is stereospecific.

32. Which of the following molecules will be the product of this substitution reaction?

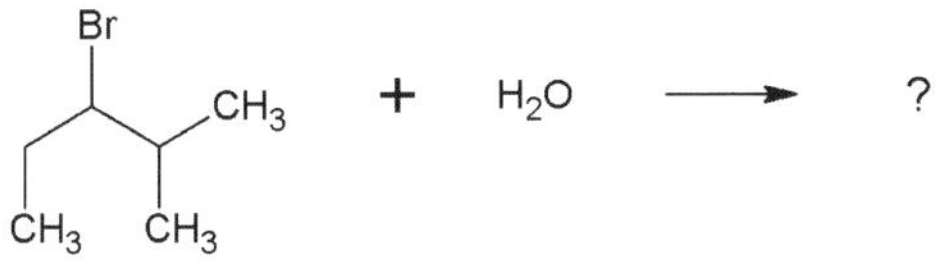

A 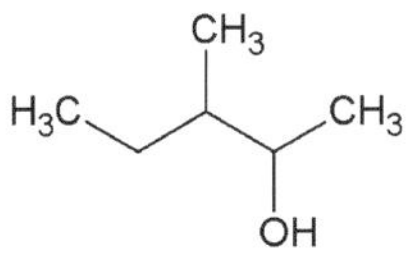

B 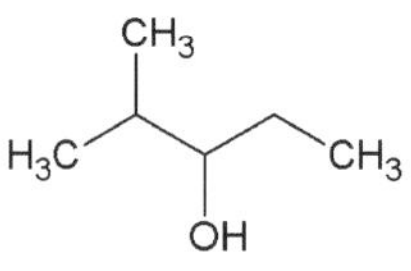

C 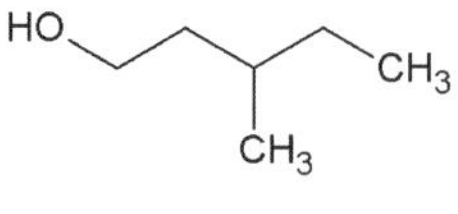

D 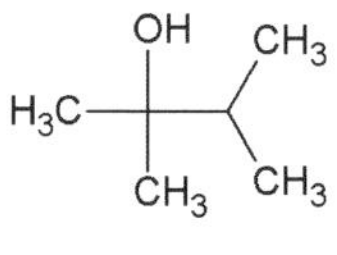

Chapter 3: Reaction Types: The GAMSAT Chemistry Challenge

33. Which of the following sets of reactants could have formed this nucleophilic substitution product?

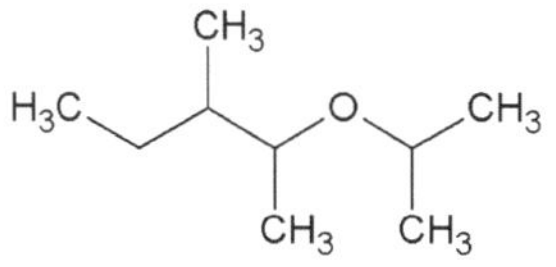

I. 2-bromo-3-methylbutane + 2-hydroxypropane (propan-2-ol)

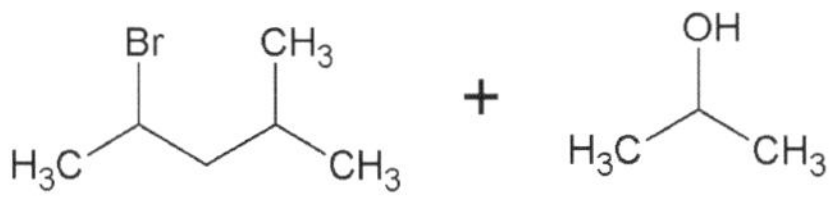

II. 3-methylbutan-2-ol + 2-bromopropane

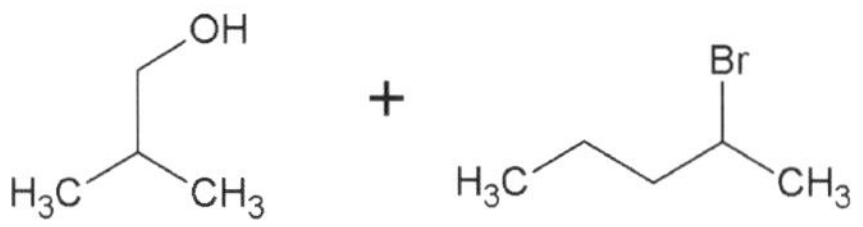

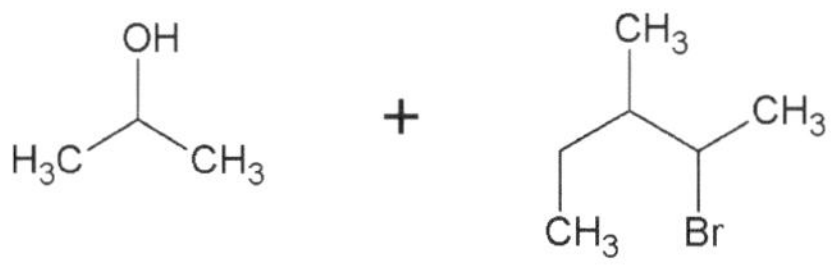

III. propan-2-ol + 2-bromo-3-methylbutane

IV. 2-bromopropane + 3-methylbutan-2-ol

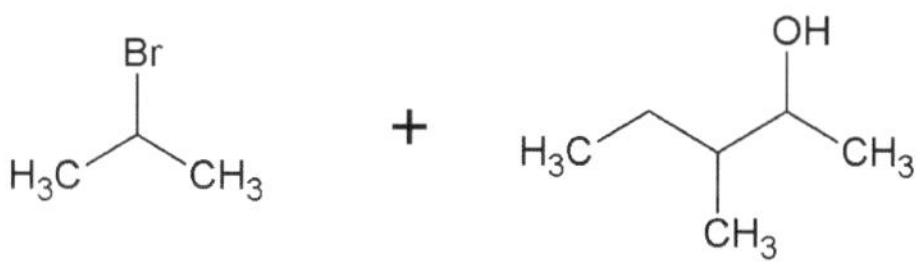

A. II only
B. I and II only
C. III and IV only
D. I, III, and IV only

Solutions

Remember to follow the 3-step method

Question 1.
   STEP 1 => What do you need to determine to solve the problem?
You need to choose the two reactants that will react to form the products given.

   STEP 2 => What relevant data provided in this problem is necessary in order to answer the question?
An example of a general transesterification reaction and the transesterification of a triglyceride with an alcohol is given in the question. Remember, the R groups represent any functional group.

   STEP 3 => Use the relevant data to solve the question
In this question, the products show that the group analogous the R" in the general reaction is $CH_3CH_2^+$, so this indicates that the alcohol in the reaction should be CH_3CH_2OH. Therefore, you know C is incorrect without further examination. The large triglyceride molecules are simply there to confuse you, but all you have to do now is compare the long carbon chains in the ethyl ester products given with the long carbon chains in the triglyceride molecules to see which ones match up. Upon comparison, the correct answer is B.

Question 2.
   STEP 1 => What do you need to determine to solve the problem?
You need to determine which molecules are esters and therefore can undergo transesterification.

   STEP 2 => What relevant data provided in this problem is necessary in order to answer the question?
The question gives you the general structure of an ester to follow, again using the R notation.

   STEP 3 => Use the relevant data to solve the question
The correct answer is D. As shown, an ester must have a carbon double bonded to an oxygen. That same carbon should have a single bond to another oxygen molecule, which is bonded to another molecule (R). Molecule II is missing an oxygen bonded to the carbon of the C=O bond. The other two molecules fit the criteria for an ester.

Chapter 3: Reaction Types: The GAMSAT Chemistry Challenge

Question 3.
STEP 1 => What do you need to determine to solve the problem?
The molecules that can catalyze a transesterification reaction.

STEP 2 => What relevant data provided in this problem is necessary in order to answer the question?
The passage tells you that an acid or a base is necessary for the catalysis of this type of reaction, and represents these as H^+ and $OR"^-$ respectively.

STEP 3 => Use the relevant data to solve the question
HCl and H_2SO_4 are both strong acids and $CH_3CH_2O^-$ is a base and thus all three can catalyze the reaction so the answer is D.

Question 4.
STEP 1 => What do you need to determine to solve the problem?
The molecule that will be a product of the given reaction.

STEP 2 => What relevant data provided in this problem is necessary in order to answer the question?
The passage gives you a general transesterification reaction to follow, replace the R, R', and R" groups in this reaction with those from the question.

STEP 3 => Use the relevant data to solve the question
As indicated in the general reaction, the result of this reaction is that the group attached to the OH of the alcohol will swap with the group attached to the O of the ester. Therefore, the CH_3CH_2 group will swap with the $CH_3CH_2CH_2$ group and the correct answer is choice A.

Question 5.
STEP 1 => What do you need to determine to solve the problem?
What molecule will be formed after rearrangement of the given structure.

STEP 2 => What relevant data provided in this problem is necessary in order to answer the question?
The passage gives you a general and specific example of a sigmatropic rearrangement that shows how the double bonds break and new bonds form in order to rearrange the molecule.

STEP 3 => Use the relevant data to solve the question
In order to solve this problem, you need to understand which bond is broken to form the cyclic intermediate and then rearrange to the new structure. In this case, the C=C bond on the side chain is broken and an intermediate cyclic compound will be created by the C from this broken bond, bonding to the ring. This will also cause the double

bonds within the ring to shift over by one carbon. In addition, the bond between the C and O on the side chain will break and a double bond will form at the end of the new side chain to compensate for the lost C-O bond. By carefully examining the original structure, pushing the bonds as described the correct structure (answer C) will be obtained.

Question 6.
STEP 1 => What do you need to determine to solve the problem?
The structure that will result after thermal hydrogen rearrangement of the molecule given.

STEP 2 => What relevant data provided in this problem is necessary in order to answer the question?
The passage gives you a general and specific example of a sigmatropic rearrangement that shows how the double bonds break and new bond form in order to rearrange the molecule.

STEP 3 => Use the relevant data to solve the question
To answer this question, again, you simply must move the bonds appropriately. In this case, the question also tells you that it will be a hydrogen shift, so, what happens is that an H from the methyl side shifts to the second carbon in the other side chain. This results in a shift of two of the double bonds, the one within the ring moves to the methyl side chain to compensate for the lost hydrogen, and the double bond in the other side chain that is closes to the ring shifts between one of the carbons within the ring and the first carbon in the side chain. Thus, the answer is A.

Question 7.
STEP 1 => What do you need to determine to solve the problem?
The number of carbons in the ring that form.

STEP 2 => What relevant data provided in this problem is necessary in order to answer the question?
The passage gives you a general and specific example of a sigmatropic rearrangement that shows how the double bonds break and new bond form in order to rearrange the molecule.

STEP 3 => Use the relevant data to solve the question
The double bond from carbon 1 will break and form a single bond between carbon 1 and 2. To compensate for the lost bond between the carbon next to carbon 1, the bond forming the three membered ring will break and shift to form a new double with the carbon next to carbon 1 thereby opening up the three membered ring and creating a larger ring. It is not even necessary at this point to worry about how the other double bonds will shift within the molecule. With the formation of the new bond between carbon 1 and 2, an 7 membered ring will now exist consisting of the newly formed ring between carbons 1 and 2 and the former three membered ring that has opened up in the rearrangement. Therefore, the answer is B.

Question 8.

STEP 1 = > **What do you need to determine to solve the problem?**
The number of double bonds that will be present in the molecule that is formed upon rearrangement.

STEP 2 = > **What relevant data provided in this problem is necessary in order to answer the question?**
By examining the examples given in the passage, they show how the double bonds break and move within the molecules.

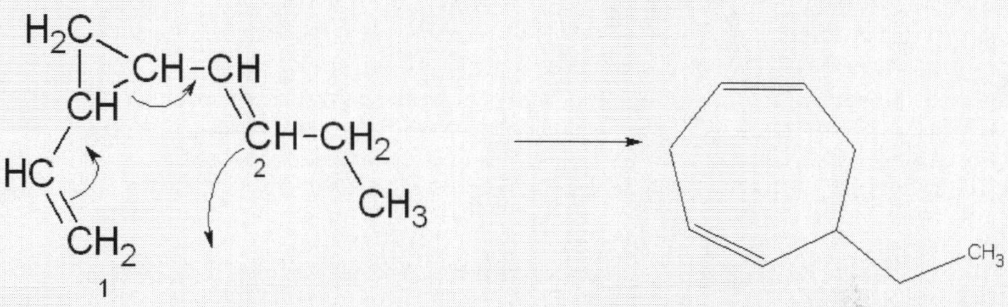

STEP 3 = > **Use the relevant data to solve the question**
As shown in the passage, the resulting molecules have the same number of bonds as the starting molecule they have simply been moved. Therefore, the correct answer is B.

Question 9.

STEP 1 = > What do you need to determine to solve the problem?
The question requires you to identify the product of the aldol condensation of a given reactant molecule.
To do so, you must know the general mechanism of the aldol reaction.

STEP 2 = > What relevant data provided in this problem is necessary in order to answer the question?
What relevant data provided in this problem is necessary in order to answer the question?
The passage indicates that the adjacent carbon of the nucleophile attacks the carbonyl carbon of the electrophile to form the new bond, which is then turned into a double bond through condensation.
This means that the carbonyl in the product must be the carbonyl of the nucleophile, and the double bond to the nucleophile must have replaced the carbonyl of the electrophile.

STEP 3 = > Use the relevant data to solve the question
Use the relevant data to solve the question
To solve the problem, you must examine each product to determine if it is the result of the reaction of the given reactant.
The nucleophile retains its structure, only replacing two hydrogen atoms from the adjacent carbon with the double bond to the electrophile. Products A, B, and C all have proper nucleophile structures, while D does not. The electrophile must also retain its carbon-chain structure, but with the new double bond to the nucleophile in place of its carbonyl group. Products A and D have the proper structure in the electrophilic portion, while B and C are the products of reactions of different electrophiles. Only Product A has the proper structure to be a product of the aldol reaction of the given reactant.

Question 10.

STEP 1 = > What do you need to determine to solve the problem?
The question requires you to identify the major product of the given aldol reaction.
All of the choices are valid products, so you must determine which one is the most favorable and is therefore the major product.

STEP 2 = > What relevant data provided in this problem is necessary in order to answer the question?
The passage indicates that in the aldol reaction, aldehydes are typically better electrophiles and ketones are typically better nucleophiles.
This means that in the given reaction, although all four given products are possible, the one with the ketone reactant forming its nucleophilic portion and the aldehyde reactant forming its electrophilic portion is the most likely to occur and is the major product.

STEP 3 = > Use the relevant data to solve the question
To solve the problem, you must determine which reactant serves as nucleophile and electrophile for each product.

The nucleophile retains it configuration in the product; therefore, Products A and B are the result of an aldol reaction with propanal as its nucleophile, while C and D are the products of an acetone nucleophile. The electrophile's structure is also retained, with the nucleophile replacing its carbonyl oxygen. Products A and C are the result of a reaction with propanal as its electrophile, while B and D are the product of an acetone electrophile. Only Product C is the result of an aldol reaction with a ketone nucleophile and an aldehyde electrophile, and is therefore the major product.

Question 11.

STEP 1 = > What do you need to determine to solve the problem?
The question requires you to identify the reactant that formed the given product in an aldol condensation.
To do so, you must determine what the structure of the product can tell you about the structure of the reactant.

STEP 2 = > What relevant data provided in this problem is necessary in order to answer the question?
The passage indicates that the carbon-carbon double bond is formed by replacing the oxygen of the electrophilic carbonyl and two hydrogen atoms from the nucleophile's adjacent carbon.
To determine the structure of the reactants that formed and aldol product, all that you have to do is "break" the carbon-carbon double bond and replace it with a carbonyl at the carbon of the electrophilic side of the bond and with two hydrogen atoms on the nucleophilic side of the bond.

STEP 3 = > Use the relevant data to solve the question
To solve the problem, you must determine the reactant that formed the given product. In this problem, only one reactant molecule was involved, as the aldol reaction occurred between two carbonyls in the same molecule, forming a cyclic product with a stable six-membered ring structure. By breaking the carbon-carbon double bond and replacing it with the original groups, the reactant obtained is Reactant D. It has the correct carbon-chain structure to produce the alkyl groups attached to the carbon ring of the product, as well as the proper spacing of the carbonyls to form a six-membered ring. While Reactant A can form a cyclohexene ring, its alkyl substituents are not properly positioned to form the given product. Reactants B and C do not have the proper structure to form the six-membered ring or its substituents, so Reactant D is the only valid reactant for the product given.

Question 12.
STEP 1 = > What do you need to determine to solve the problem?
The question requires you to determine which of the given reactants can undergo both steps of the aldol reaction. To do so, you must understand what is necessary for the aldol reaction to occur.

STEP 2 = > What relevant data provided in this problem is necessary in order to answer the question?
The passage indicates that the aldol addition is characterized by the nucleophile's adjacent carbon losing an electron and reducing the electrophile's carbonyl.
The aldol condensation then results in the loss of another hydrogen atom from the nucleophilic carbon of the new bond and the addition product's alcohol in favor of a double bond. The key is that to proceed completely through both steps requires the nucleophile to have at least two hydrogen atoms on the same carbon adjacent to the carbonyl.

STEP 3 = > Use the relevant data to solve the question
To solve the problem, you must examine the structure of each reactant to determine if it is capable of undergoing aldol addition and condensation with itself.
Since each reactant would have to serve as both electrophile and nucleophile in a reaction with itself, the important thing to look for is the presence of two hydrogen atoms on the same carbon adjacent to the carbonyl, a requirement for a molecule to serve as an aldol nucleophile. Reactant A, 2-methylpropanal, has only one hydrogen atom in the proper position, and can therefore serve as a nucleophile for aldol addition but not aldol condensation. Reactant B, benzaldehyde, has no adjacent hydrogen atoms and cannot serve as an aldol nucleophile at all. Reactant C, 3-methylbutanone, has only one hydrogen atom on the interior adjacent carbon, but has three on the terminal carbon and can therefore undergo both aldol addition and aldol condensation with the terminal carbon as its nucleophile. Reactant D, 2-methylpentanal, is chemically similar to Reactant A for the purposes of the aldol reaction in that its lone adjacent hydrogen atom will only allow it to undergo aldol addition, not aldol condensation. Only Reactant C has the proper carbon-chain structure to allow it to function as both nucleophile and electrophile in a complete aldol reaction.

Question 13.
STEP 1 = > What do you need to determine to solve the problem?
The question requires you to determine which of the given molecules can be produced in an aldol reaction.
To do so, you must identify the general characteristics of aldol products and compare them to the given products.

STEP 2 = > What relevant data provided in this problem is necessary in order to answer the question?
The passage indicates that the aldol addition reaction results in a carbonyl compound with an alcohol group bonded to the second carbon down the chain from the carbonyl carbon.

The aldol condensation product is a carbonyl compound with a double bond between the first and second carbons adjacent to the carbonyl group.

STEP 3 = > Use the relevant data to solve the question
To solve the problem, each given product must be compared to the template for aldol products.
Product I has an alcohol group, but it is on the first carbon adjacent to the carbonyl instead of the second carbon, so it is not an aldol product. Product II has a carbon-carbon double bond, but it is between the second and third carbons from the carbonyl, not the first and second, so it is not an aldol product. Product III has an alcohol group bonded to the second carbon from the carbonyl, and is an aldol addition product. Product IV has a double bond between the first and second carbons from the carbonyl, and is an aldol condensation product. Therefore, only Products III and IV are aldol products.

Question 14.

STEP 1 = > What do you need to determine to solve the problem?
The question requires you to identify the molecule with a specific oxidation number for chlorine.
To do so, you must calculate the oxidation numbers for each molecule.

STEP 2 = > What relevant data provided in this problem is necessary in order to answer the question?
The passage indicates that the total of the oxidation numbers of a molecule or ion is its charge.
Also, the charge on oxygen in a polyatomic structure is typically -2.

STEP 3 = > Use the relevant data to solve the question
The total oxidation number for each molecule must be zero, as all are neutral.
Since each cation is sodium, which can only have an oxidation number of +1, the oxidation number of the chlorine-containing anions must all be -1. The Cl- chloride ion is simple; its oxidation number is -1. In chlorite, ClO_2^-, the chlorine oxidation number must be +3 to balance the -2 from each oxygen atom. In chlorate, ClO_3^-, the chlorine oxidation number must be +5 to balance the oxygen numbers; in perchlorate, ClO_4^-, the chlorine oxidation number is +7. Therefore, chlorate is the correct answer.

Question 15.
   STEP 1 = > What do you need to determine to solve the problem?
   The question requires that you identify which element is reduced in the given reaction. To do so, you must calculate the oxidation states for each element before and after the reaction.

   STEP 2 = > What relevant data provided in this problem is necessary in order to answer the question?
   The passage indicates that the oxidation sate of an ion is equal to its charge; for the metals, this means that their charge is their oxidation state as they are single-atom cations.
   Also, the passage indicates that the species that is reduced gains electrons and its oxidation number becomes more negative.

   STEP 3 = > Use the relevant data to solve the question
   The oxidation state on sulfur and chlorine is unchanged from reactants to products. The oxidation state of silver changes from +1 to +2, and the oxidation number of copper goes from +2 to +1. Since the oxidation number of copper went down, it is the species that is reduced.

Question 16.
   STEP 1 = > What do you need to determine to solve the problem?
   The question requires you to identify the reducing agent from the same reaction as the previous question.
   To do so, you must determine what a reducing agent does.

   STEP 2 = > What relevant data provided in this problem is necessary in order to answer the question?
   The passage indicates that the reducing agent is the species that gives up electrons, allowing another species to be reduced and becoming oxidized itself.

   STEP 3 = > Use the relevant data to solve the question
   Since you have already calculated the oxidation states from the previous problem, it is a simple matter to identify silver as the element that is oxidized.
   This means that the reducing agent is the molecule that contains silver on the reactant side, which is silver chloride. Copper sulfate is the oxidizing agent, while silver sulfate and copper chloride are the products and are not either agent.

Question 17.

STEP 1 = > What do you need to determine to solve the problem?
What do you need to determine to solve the problem?
The question requires you to identify the redox reaction from among the choices.
To do so, you must first understand what a redox reaction is.

STEP 2 = > What relevant data provided in this problem is necessary in order to answer the question?
What relevant data provided in this problem is necessary in order to answer the question?
The passage indicates that a redox reaction is one in which the oxidation states of some species change as electrons are passed between atoms.

STEP 3 = > Use the relevant data to solve the question
As all of the reactions are between common and fairly simple ions, it is rather easy to see that the charges, and therefore the oxidation states, of the elements are unchanged in the first three reactions.
However, in the fourth reaction, an electron is passed from cobalt to titanium, making it a redox reaction.

Question 18.

STEP 1 = > What do you need to determine to solve the problem?
The question requires you to identify the amount of electrons passed between lead and iron during the given reaction.
To do so, you must understand how a redox reaction works.

STEP 2 = > What relevant data provided in this problem is necessary in order to answer the question?
The passage indicates that both oxidation and reduction are processes in which electrons are transferred.
Also, in the typical redox reaction both are occurring simultaneously, each facilitating the other. For each increment that the oxidation number of a species changes, one electron has been transferred.

STEP 3 = > Use the relevant data to solve the question
The oxidation number of the iron atom changes from 0 to +2 during the reaction, which means that 2 electrons have been transferred.
Therefore, for every mole of metallic iron that is consumed, 2 moles of electrons will be transferred to lead.

Question 19.
STEP 1 = > What do you need to determine to solve the problem?
The question requires you to identify the antiaromatic structures in the diagrams.
To do so, you must determine what makes a molecule antiaromatic.

STEP 2 = > What relevant data provided in this problem is necessary in order to answer the question?
The passage indicates that aromaticity and antiaromaticity is based on electrons in π-orbitals. Ring structures with conjugated double bonds, lone pairs, or ionized orbitals can form aromatic molecules by overlapping p-orbitals. In rings of this nature, aromatic molecules are the ones with an odd number of electron pairs in the π system, while antiaromatic rings have an even number of contributing electron pairs.

STEP 3 = > Use the relevant data to solve the question
Each of the molecules shown has an aromatic π-ring, formed of double bonds and the unbonded p-orbital of the charged atom.
Each of the cyclopropene rings has a single electron pair in double bonding, while the cyclopentadiene rings have two pairs in double bonds. Each of the anions has an additional pair in its unbonded p-orbital, while the cations have an empty orbital that can conjugate but cannot contribute electrons. Therefore, Choices I and IV have two electron pairs in the π system, while Choice II has one and Choice III has three. II and III are aromatic, while I and IV are antiaromatic.

Question 20.
STEP 1 = > What do you need to determine to solve the problem?
The question requires you to identify the more reactive lone pair between the two heterocyclic molecules.
To do so, you must determine what the relevant influence on reactivity is.

STEP 2 = > What relevant data provided in this problem is necessary in order to answer the question?
The passage indicates that lone pairs can participate in aromaticity.
Also, the passage indicates that aromaticity is dependent on the number of π electrons in the rings.

STEP 3 = > Use the relevant data to solve the question
Molecule A has two double bonds, so to complete the conjugation and achieve the correct number of electrons for aromaticity, its nitrogen lone pair must participate in aromaticity. Therefore, Choice B is factually incorrect. Molecule B has three conjugated double bonds in its six-membered ring, so it has benzene character and is aromatic without using its nitrogen lone pair. Therefore, Choice C is factually incorrect. Furthermore, Molecule A's lone pair is tied up in the aromatic structure, while Molecule B's lone pair is projecting in an unbonded orbital away from the ring and is much more available for reaction. Therefore, Choice D is the correct answer.

Question 21.
   STEP 1 = > What do you need to determine to solve the problem?
   The question requires you to identify the least stable of the molecules given.
   To do so, you must determine what effect aromaticity has on stability.

   STEP 2 = > What relevant data provided in this problem is necessary in order to answer the question?
   The passage indicates that aromatic rings are highly stable compared to their saturated counterparts, while antiaromatic molecules are highly destabilized.

   STEP 3 = > Use the relevant data to solve the question
   Choice C is a ring with 6 conjugated π electrons, Choice A is a ring structure with 10 conjugated π electrons, and Choice D is a ring structure with 14 conjugated π electrons. All of these molecules are aromatic and highly stable. However, Choice B does not have a fully conjugated π system, and therefore does not have the same aromatic character as the others. It is the least stable of the molecules due to its lack of complete aromaticity.

Question 22.
   STEP 1 = > What do you need to determine to solve the problem?
   The question requires you to identify the aromatic structures in the diagrams.
   To do so, you must determine what makes a molecule aromatic.

   STEP 2 = > What relevant data provided in this problem is necessary in order to answer the question?
   The passage indicates that aromaticity and antiaromaticity is based on electrons in π-orbitals. Ring structures with conjugated double bonds, lone pairs, or ionized orbitals can form aromatic molecules by overlapping p-orbitals. In rings of this nature, aromatic molecules are the ones with an odd number of electron pairs in the π system, while antiaromatic rings have an even number of contributing electron pairs.

   STEP 3 = > Use the relevant data to solve the question
   Each of the molecules has the conjugated π bonding ring necessary for aromatic character. Molecule I has two π electron pairs in the ring, Molecule II has three π electron pairs, Molecule III has four π electron pairs, and Molecule IV has five π electron pairs. According to the rules of aromaticity, II and IV are aromatic while I and III are antiaromatic, so Choice B is correct.

Question 23.
STEP 1 = > What do you need to determine to solve the problem?
The question requires you to identify the least stressful bond angle in an aromatic ring.
To do so, you must determine what the optimum geometry of an aromatic structure is.

STEP 2 = > What relevant data provided in this problem is necessary in order to answer the question?
The passage indicates that aromaticity is characterized by a planar ring with a single perpendicular π orbital on each atom in the ring contributing to the aromatic bond.

STEP 3 = > Use the relevant data to solve the question
The indicated geometry suggests that the ideal bond hybridization pattern for an aromatic ring is sp2, with an unhybridized p orbital for aromaticity.
Therefore, the optimum bond angle for an aromatic structure is 120°.

Question 24.
STEP 1 = > What do you need to determine to solve the problem?
The question requires you to identify the product of the given reaction.
To do so, you must understand the process of the Diels-Alder reaction.

STEP 2 = > What relevant data provided in this problem is necessary in order to answer the question?
The passage indicates that the diene and dienophile react as shown in the passage diagram, forming a new cyclohexene ring with substitution patterns related to the structure of the reactants as shown.

STEP 3 = > Use the relevant data to solve the question

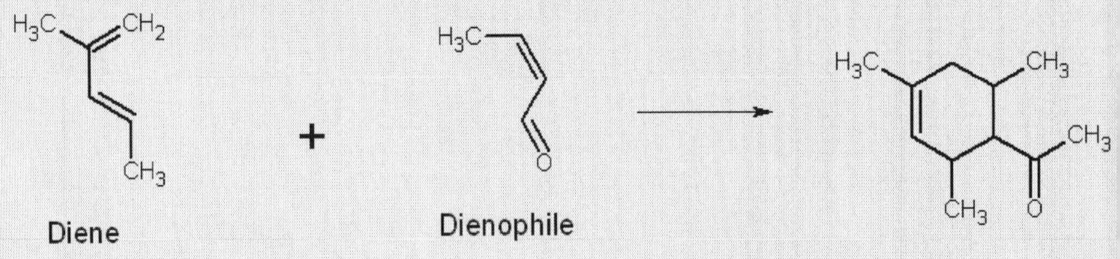

The structure of the Diels-Alder product can be determined from the reactants by orienting the molecules correctly and joining the diene and dienophile in the pattern shown in the passage diagram.

When the product choices are examined, all have the acetyl group correctly positioned, but only D has all three methyl groups in appropriate locations.

Chapter 3: Reaction Types: The GAMSAT Chemistry Challenge

Question 25.
STEP 1 = > What do you need to determine to solve the problem?
The question requires you to identify which molecule is the product of the reaction of a Diels-Alder product.
To do so, you must determine what the reactants were for each product.

STEP 2 = > What relevant data provided in this problem is necessary in order to answer the question?
The passage indicates that the Diels-Alder product is a cyclohexene with the double bond on the side opposite the dienophile portion of the structure.

STEP 3 = > Use the relevant data to solve the question
For one of the reactants that formed the product to be a Diels-Alder product, it must have been the dienophile in the reaction.
Therefore, the product must be a bicyclic structure with the double bond on one cyclohexene ring directly opposite the second cyclohexane ring. Only Product B has the correct structure to be the product of the reaction of a Diels-Alder product.

Question 26.
STEP 1 = > What do you need to determine to solve the problem?
The question requires you to identify the possible reactant pairs for the given product. To do so, you must determine where the product's substituents could have originated.

STEP 2 = > What relevant data provided in this problem is necessary in order to answer the question?
The passage indicates that the product of a reaction with an alkyne dienophile is a cyclohexadiene ring, with the double bonds opposite one another.

STEP 3 = > Use the relevant data to solve the question
In the product shown, either of the double bonds could be the dienophile remnant, which means that either two substituents came from each the diene and dienophile, or all four came from the diene.
Only Reactant Pair IV has the appropriate structures to satisfy the first case, and only Reactant Pair II is correct for the second. Therefore, Choice C is correct.

Question 27.
STEP 1 = > What do you need to determine to solve the problem?
The question requires you to determine the number of possible Diels-Alder products of the reaction of the given reactant with itself.
To do so, you must understand what the possible reactions are.

STEP 2 = > What relevant data provided in this problem is necessary in order to answer the question?
The passage indicates that the Diels-Alder reaction can take place between any conjugated diene and a dienophile, any multiple bond.

STEP 3 = > Use the relevant data to solve the question
There is only one possible diene in the reactant, but it can react with either of the two double bonds as dienophiles, and each reaction can proceed through two orientations, for a total of four possible products.

Question 28.
STEP 1 = > What do you need to determine to solve the problem?
The question requires you to identify the major product of the shown reaction. To do so you must determine what the most favorable product arrangement is.

STEP 2 = > What relevant data provided in this problem is necessary in order to answer the question?
The passage indicates that 1,2- and 1,4- substituted products are more favorable than 1,3- substituted products.

STEP 3 = > Use the relevant data to solve the question
Products B and D have impossible structures for the given reaction.
Products A and C have possible structures, but Product C is 1,3-substituted while Product A is 1,4-substituted; therefore, Product A is the major product.

Question 29.
STEP 1 = > What do you need to determine to solve the problem?
The question requires you to identify the SN2 product of the reaction shown. To do so, you must determine what the characteristics of an SN2 reaction are.

STEP 2 = > What relevant data provided in this problem is necessary in order to answer the question?
The passage indicates that the SN2 reaction is the replacement of a leaving group with a nucleophile, with an inversion of stereochemistry at a chiral center.

STEP 3 = > Use the relevant data to solve the question
In the reaction shown, the bromine atoms serve as the leaving group and the water molecules serve as the nucleophile, forming alcohols.
Both substituents are located at chiral carbons, so the stereochemistry of each will invert. This means that both substituent bonds must flip through the plane of the diagram; therefore Product C is the correct structure.

Question 30.
STEP 1 = > What do you need to determine to solve the problem?
The question requires you to identify the most likely substitution mechanism for the reaction shown.
To do so, you must understand the differences between the two mechanisms.

STEP 2 = > What relevant data provided in this problem is necessary in order to answer the question?
The passage indicates that the primary difference between the two mechanisms is that S_N1 proceeds through a carbocation transition state and produces a racemic mixture, while S_N2 involves a rear attack, proceeds through a pentacoordinate intermediate, and results in an inversion of stereochemistry.

STEP 3 = > Use the relevant data to solve the question
The reactant shown is a tertiary alkyl halide, with bulky alkyl groups that sterically inhibit the nucleophile from attacking the carbon in S_N2 fashion. Therefore, the expected mechanism is S_N1, due to steric hindrance of the alkyl halide.

Question 31.
STEP 1 = > What do you need to determine to solve the problem?
The question requires you to identify the mechanism of a substitution reaction based on its product.
To do so, you must understand what products each mechanism yields.

STEP 2 = > What relevant data provided in this problem is necessary in order to answer the question?
The passage indicates that the primary difference between the two mechanisms is that SN1 proceeds through a carbocation transition state and produces a racemic mixture, while SN2 involves a rear attack, proceeds through a pentacoordinate intermediate, and results in an inversion of stereochemistry.

STEP 3 = > Use the relevant data to solve the question
Use the relevant data to solve the question
The product given is stereospecific at its chiral center, and is by far the dominant product. The product is not a racemic mixture, and is therefore the product of an SN2 reaction, as evidenced by stereoselectivity.

Question 32.
STEP 1 = > What do you need to determine to solve the problem?
The question requires you to identify the product of a general substitution reaction. To do

so, you must determine what the general characteristics of a substitution reaction are.

STEP 2 => What relevant data provided in this problem is necessary in order to answer the question?
The passage indicates that a substitution reaction replaces a leaving group with a nucleophile, preserving the structure of the reactant's carbon chain.

STEP 3 => Use the relevant data to solve the question
In this reaction, the bromine serves as the leaving group, while the war nucleophile forms an alcohol substituent on the product.
The product must be identical to the reactant except for the alcohol in place of the bromine. Products A, C, and D all have incorrect structures, but Product B has the correct configuration to be the product of the reaction.

Question 33.
STEP 1 => What do you need to determine to solve the problem?
The question requires you to identify the reactant pairs that could form the substitution product shown.
To do so, you must determine what the structure of a substitution product reveals about the reactants.

STEP 2 => What relevant data provided in this problem is necessary in order to answer the question?
The passage indicates that a substitution reaction replaces a leaving group with a nucleophile, preserving the structure of the reactant's carbon chain.

STEP 3 => Use the relevant data to solve the question
In this reaction, a bromine atom is the leaving group, while an alcohol nucleophile replaces it to form an ether.
The substitution mechanism means that the carbon chains on each side of the ether could have been either the alkyl halide or the alcohol, but the carbon structure of the reactants must be preserved in the product. Reactant Pairs I and II have incorrect carbon-chain structures for the product given. Reactant Pairs III and IV have the correct structures, with the only difference being the location of the bromide and alcohol groups. Therefore, Choice C is correct.

CHAPTER 4: **Isomerism**

Key Concept: Isomerism

Different compounds that have the same molecular formula are called isomers. These compounds will contain the same kinds and numbers of atoms, but the atoms will be connected to one another in different ways. Isomers are different compounds because they have different molecular structures, and the structural differences result in different properties. The difference in structure and properties can be so great that the isomers are assigned to different families, i.e. ethyl alcohol and dimethyl ether (C_2H_6O).

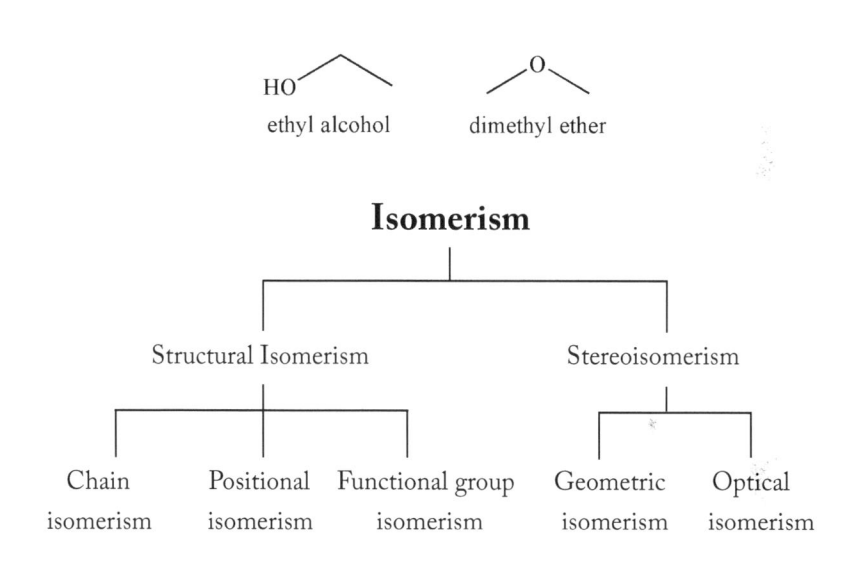

HO‾\‾   ‾\‾O‾\‾
ethyl alcohol   dimethyl ether

Isomerism
- Structural Isomerism
  - Chain isomerism
  - Positional isomerism
  - Functional group isomerism
- Stereoisomerism
  - Geometric isomerism
  - Optical isomerism

Key Concepts: Structural Isomerism

In structural isomerism, the atoms are arranged in a different order. In other words, these molecules, like all isomers have the same molecular formula, but are connected to each other in different ways. There are three types of structural isomers, chain isomers, positional isomers, and functional group isomers.

Chain Isomerism

This type of isomer arises because of the possibility of branching within the carbon chain. It is quite easy to see this in alkanes. For example, butane C_4H_{10} has two possible arrangements. In one, the carbon atoms lie in a straight chain, where as with the other, the chain has a branch.

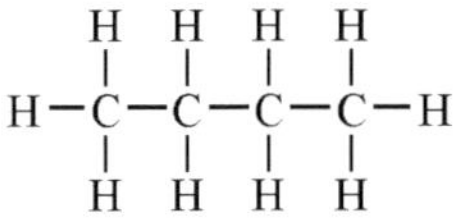

```
H H H H                    H H H
| | | |                    | | |
H-C-C-C-C-H            H-C-C-C-H
| | | |                    | | |
H H H H                    H C H
                              / | \
                             H  |  H
                                H
```

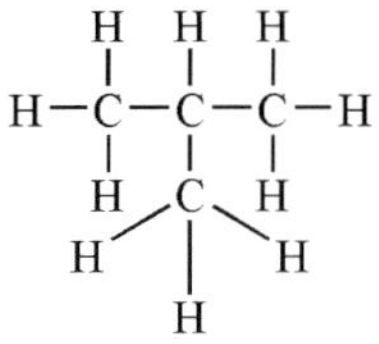

butane   methylpropane
b.p. 273K   b.p. 261K

One important thing to note is that you need to be very careful not to confuse "false" isomers which are simply twisted versions of the original molecule with real isomers. For example, butane shown below is just the straight chain configuration rotated about the central atom.

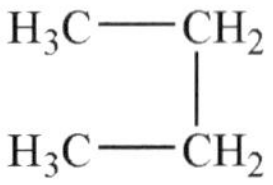

```
H₃C ── CH₂
        |
H₃C ── CH₂
```

As the number of carbon atoms increase, the number of possible isomers increases exponentially

Formula	Number of structural isomers
C_5H_{12}	3
C_6H_{14}	5
C_7H_{16}	9
$C_{10}H_{22}$	75
$C_{20}H_{42}$	366319
$C_{30}H_{62}$	Over 4 billion

Positional Isomers

This occurs when isomers have the same carbon skeleton, but important groups are placed in different positions within the molecule. i.e. same molecular formula, different structural formula. With these isomers, it would be impossible to twist one isomer to turn it onto another isomer.

Two examples are shown below.

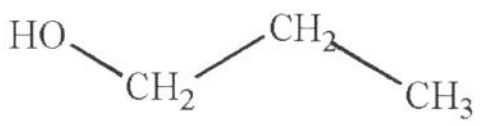

propan-1-ol

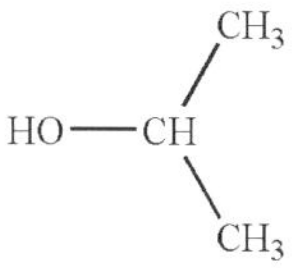

propan-2-ol

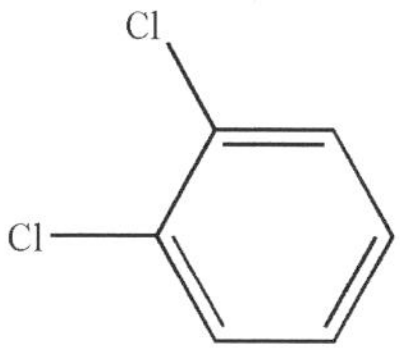

1,2-dichlorobenzene

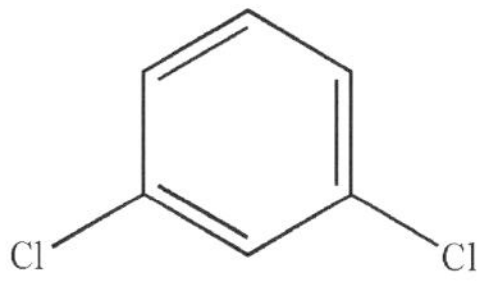

1,3-dichlorobenzene

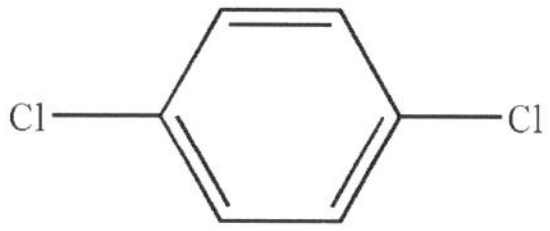

1,4-dichlorobenzene

Functional Group Isomers

In this type of structural isomer, the isomers contain different functional groups, meaning they belong to different families of compounds. For example, lets examine the molecular formula C_3H_6O.

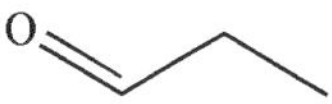

propanal

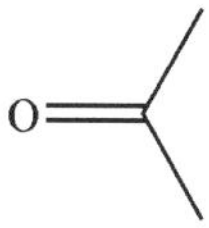

propanone

You can get an aldehyde (propanal) or a ketone (propanone) from this formula. There are other possibilites as well, however we won't list them all here. Another example is the molecular formula $C_4H_8O_2$. Two of the possible isomers of this molecular formula are a carboxylic acid and an ester, shown below.

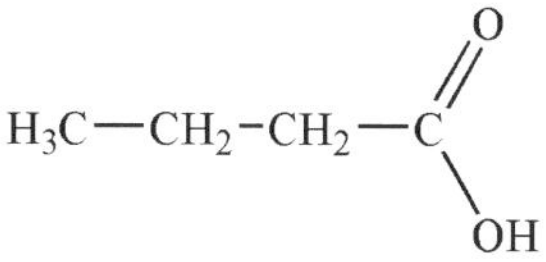

Butyric acid

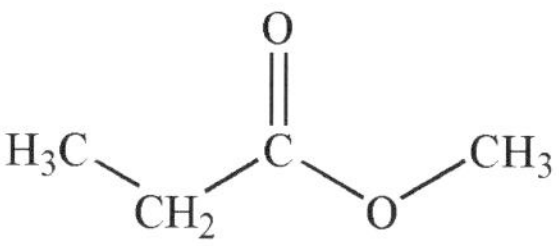

methyl butanoate

Key Concept: Stereoisomerism

Stereoisomers have identical molecular formulae, and the atoms are linked together in the same order, but have different 3 dimensional.

The two types of stereoisomerism are
- Geometric (or cis-trans) isomerism
- Optical isomerism

---> Quick Facts: Geometrical Isomerism

- A form of **stereoisomerism**.
- Found in alkenes.
- Occurs due to the **restricted rotation of C=C double bonds.**
- Doesn't occur with **single bonds** because they can **rotate.**
- The two forms are known as **CIS** and **TRANS.**
- Doesn't occur when two similar groups/atoms are on the same end of the double bond.

Geometric isomerism exists because the π bond of the C=C bond prevents free rotation. Below are examples of geometric isomers of dichloromethane and butenedioic acid

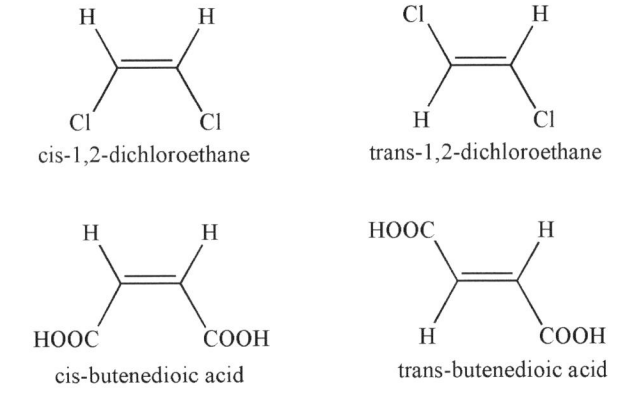

cis-1,2-dichloroethane

trans-1,2-dichloroethane

cis-butenedioic acid

trans-butenedioic acid

Key Concept: Optical Isomerism

Examine your left and right hand. They are mirror images of each other and you can not superimpose them on top of each other so that each finger coincides with the identical finger on the opposite hand. In addition, a right hand glove will not fit on the left hand and visa versa. Hands have no plane of symmetry, centre of symmetry, or axis of symmetry. Just like your hands

Chapter 4: Isomerism

many chemical compounds can exist in two mirror forms. Optical isomers arise when there is no symmetry in the molecule, thus the molecule is called asymmetric. Chirality is the key to optical isomers and arises from asymmetry. Carbon atoms can have four single bonds and these bonds are arranged tetrahedrally (pyramid shape).

When there are four different atoms attached to the carbon, it is a chiral carbon.

–>Quick Facts: Optical Isomerism

- A form of stereoisomerism.
- The different forms are known as **optical isomers** or **enantiomers.**
- Occurs when compounds have an **asymmetric carbon atom.**
- Occurs when compounds have **4 different groups attached to the same carbon.**
- **TWO** isomers that are **non-superimposable mirror images** of each other.
- One isomer rotates light to the right DEXTROROTATORY; D or (+).
- The other rotates light to the left LAEVOROTATORY ; L or (-).
- Rotation of light is measured using a polarimeter.
- Rotation is measured by observing the polarised light coming towards the observer.
- A 50/50 mixture of the two enantiomers is a racemic mixture.

The diagram below shows the optical isomers of lactic acid and glyceraldehydes.

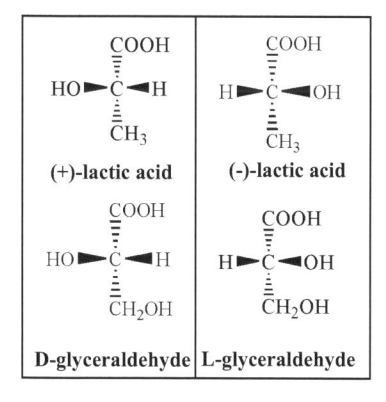

(+)-lactic acid	(-)-lactic acid
HO—C—H, COOH above, CH$_3$ below	H—C—OH, COOH above, CH$_3$ below
D-glyceraldehyde	L-glyceraldehyde
HO—C—H, COOH above, CH$_2$OH below	H—C—OH, COOH above, CH$_2$OH below

Practice Questions

Question (1-4).

When migration of a proton from a carbon atom to the adjacent carbon atom occurs, the two forms are found to be in dynamic equilibrium with each other. The enol tautomer is formed by the transfer of an acid hydrogen from the alpha carbon to the carbonyl oxygen.

1. The enol form of acetoacetic acid ($CH_3COHCHCOOH$) contains
   A. 12 σ bonds, 2π bonds, 4 lone pair of electrons
   B. 11 σ bonds, 2π bonds, 6 lone pair of electrons
   C. 10 σ bonds, 2π bonds, 6 lone pair of electrons
   D. 12 σ bonds, 3π bonds, 4 lone pair of electrons

2. The correct order of increasing enol content is
   A. $CH_3CHO<CH_3COCH_3<CH_3COCH_2COCH_3<CH_3COCH_2CH_2COOH$
   B. $CH_3CHO<CH_3COCH_2CH_2COOH<CH_3COCH_3<CH_3COCH_2COCH_3$
   C. $CH_3CHO<CH_3COCH_3<CH_3COCH_2CH_2COOH<CH_3COCH_2COCH_3$
   D. $CH_3COCH_2CH_2COOH<CH_3CHO<CH_3COCH_3<CH_3COCH_2COCH_3$

3. The enolic form of acetone (CH_3COCH_3) contains

	σ bonds	π bonds	lone pair of electrons
A.	8	1	2
B.	8	2	2
C.	10	1	1
D.	9	2	1

4. Primary alcohols are compounds containing – CH_2OH group. How many isomers of $C_5H_{11}OH$ will be primary alcohols?
   A. 2
   B. 3
   C. 4
   D. 5

Question (5-9).

The requirements of geometric isomerism in alkenes are,
1. The presence of a π bond
2. Each π bonded carbon should be attached to two unlike groups.

When the like groups are on the same plane it is called a cis- isomer and when like groups are on the opposite side of the plane, it's called a trans- isomer.

5. Each of the following compounds shows geometrical isomerism EXCEPT
    A. 2-pentene
    B. 2-methyl-2-pentene
    C. 2-butene
    D. 3-methyl-3-hexene

6. Which of the following can exist as cis-and trans isomers?
    A. $CH_2=CHCl$
    B. $CH_2=CH-CH=CH_2$
    C. $CH_3CH_2CH=CHCl$
    D. $CHCl=CCl_2$

7. Which one of the following compounds will show geometrical isomerism?

    A. 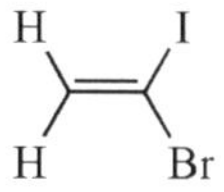 H, H / I, Br
    B. 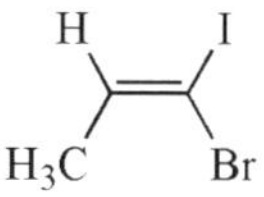 H, H$_3$C / I, Br
    C. 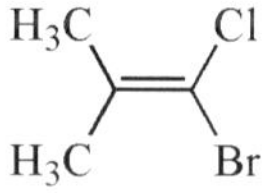 H$_3$C, H$_3$C / Cl, Br
    D. 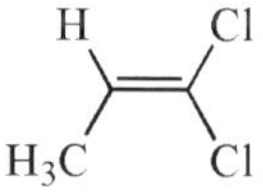 H, H$_3$C / Cl, Cl

8. The number of geometrical isomers in case of a compound with the structure $CH_3-CH=CH-CH=CH-C_2H_5$ is
    A. 2
    B. 3
    C. 4
    D. 5

9. The following structure is a ?

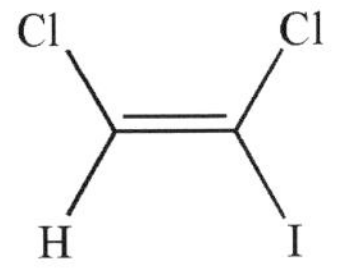

$$\underset{H}{\overset{Cl}{>}}C=C\underset{I}{\overset{Cl}{<}}$$

A. A cis-isomer
B. A trans-isomer
C. Racemic mixture
D. None

Solution

Question 1
The enol form of Acetoacetic acid formula is

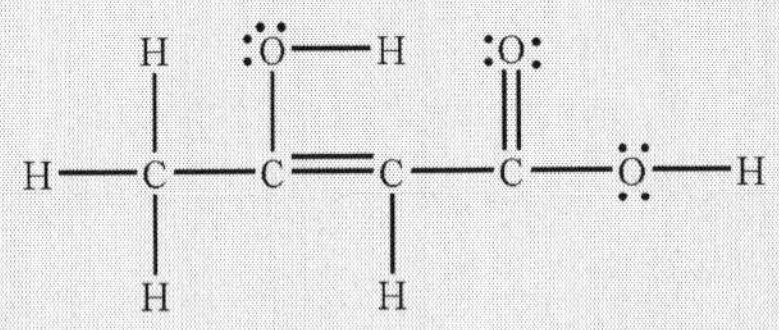

$$H-\underset{H}{\overset{H}{C}}-C=C-C-\ddot{O}-H$$
(with OH on second C and =O on fourth C)

It contains 11σ, 2π bonds and 6 lone pair of electrons. The correct answer is B.

Question 2
As the acidic strength of α–hydrogen in aldehydes/ketones increases, the rate of enol formation increases. This change of keto into enol form is therefore also dependant on the presence of an electron withdrawing group and stabilization of the anion.

The conjugate base of acetone is more resonance stabilized than the conjugate base of acetaldehyde. Therefore CH_3COCH_3 will have higher enol content than CH_3CHO. An electron-withdrawing group is present on $CH_3COCH_2CH_2COCH_3$. Due to presence of the e- withdrawing group acidity increases and thus the rate of enol formation increases. An electron-withdrawing group is also present on $CH_3COCH_2CH_2COOH$ but at the β – position. The correct order of enol content is given in answer C.

Question 3

The enol form of acetone, CH_3COCH_3 is,

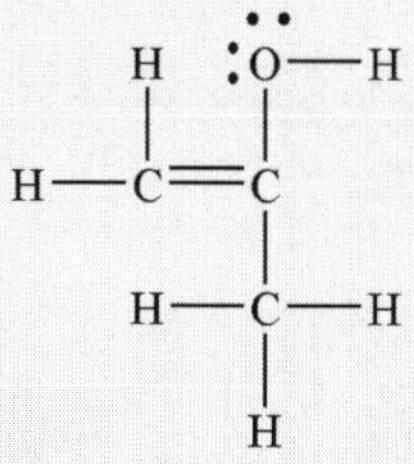

```
        H   :Ö—H
        |   |
    H—C===C
        |
    H—C—H
        |
        H
```

Because it is in the enol form, the double bond will be between the two carbons instead of having a C=O, which would be the keto form.
It contains 8 σ bonds, 1 π bond and two lone pairs of electron. This combination is given in answer A.

Question 4

Alcohols are the compounds containing – CH_2OH group. The isomers of $C_5H_{11}OH$ are

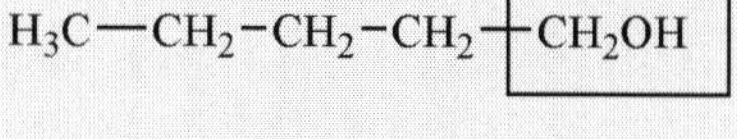

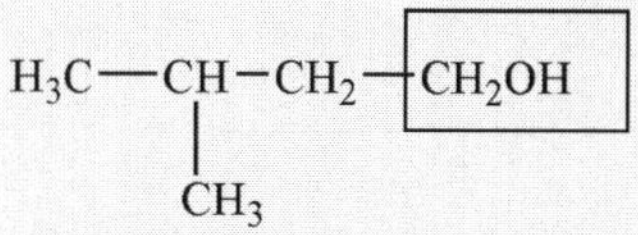

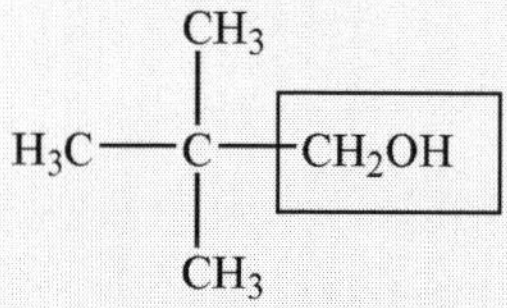

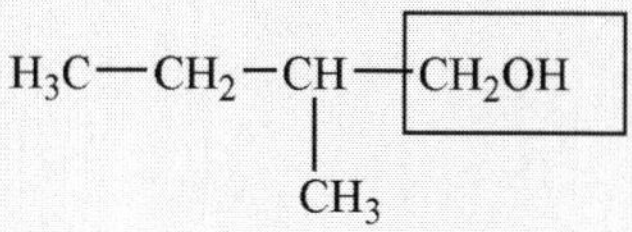

$H_3C-CH_2-CH_2-CH_2-\boxed{CH_2OH}$

$H_3C-CH-CH_2-\boxed{CH_2OH}$
$\qquad\quad |$
$\qquad\;\, CH_3$

$\qquad\quad CH_3$
$\qquad\quad\; |$
$H_3C-C-\boxed{CH_2OH}$
$\qquad\quad\; |$
$\qquad\quad CH_3$

$H_3C-CH_2-CH-\boxed{CH_2OH}$
$\qquad\qquad\quad |$
$\qquad\qquad\; CH_3$

There are four primary alcohols; the answer is C.

Question 5

The conditions for a molecule to show geometrical isomerism are

  i) The presence of π bond

  ii) Two unlike groups present at each double bonded carbon.

The only molecule which does not satisfy these conditions is 2-methyl-2-pentene, because it has two methyl groups on C_2, answer B.

Question 6

The compound in answer C show geometrical isomerism

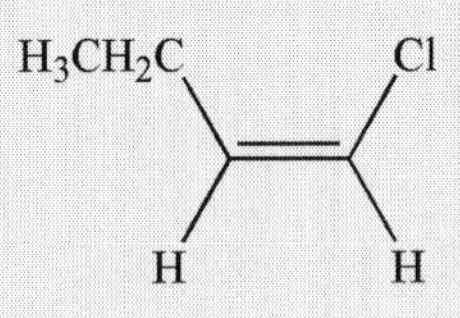

$$\underset{\text{cis}}{\begin{array}{c}H_3CH_2C\\H\end{array}\!\!\!\!\diagup\!\!\!=\!\!\!\diagdown\!\!\!\!\begin{array}{c}Cl\\H\end{array}} \qquad \underset{\text{trans}}{\begin{array}{c}H_3CH_2C\\H\end{array}\!\!\!\!\diagup\!\!\!=\!\!\!\diagdown\!\!\!\!\begin{array}{c}H\\Cl\end{array}}$$

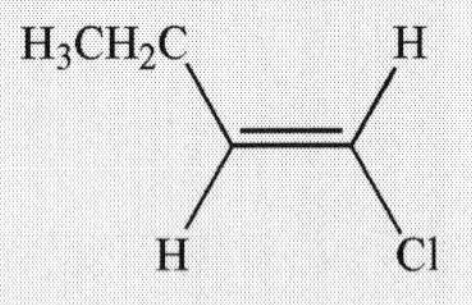

Question 7

Only the compound in answer B can show geometrical isomerism

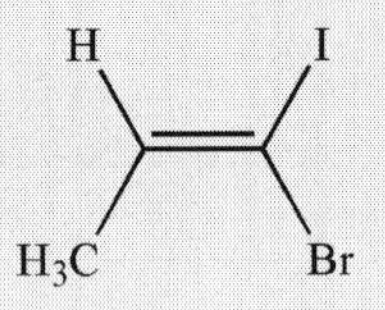

$$\underset{\text{trans}}{\begin{array}{c}H\\H_3C\end{array}\!\!\!\!\diagup\!\!\!=\!\!\!\diagdown\!\!\!\!\begin{array}{c}I\\Br\end{array}} \qquad \underset{\text{cis}}{\begin{array}{c}H\\H_3C\end{array}\!\!\!\!\diagup\!\!\!=\!\!\!\diagdown\!\!\!\!\begin{array}{c}Br\\I\end{array}}$$

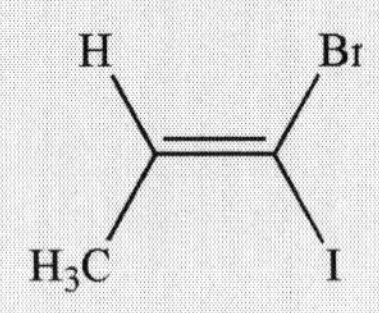

Question 8

These are four geometrical isomers, answer C.

[Structure 1: H₃C and CH=CHC₂H₅ on top; H and H on bottom of C=C]

[Structure 2: H₃C and H on top; H and CH=CHC₂H₅ on bottom of C=C]

[Structure 3: H₃CHC=CH and C₂H₅ on top; H and H on bottom of C=C]

[Structure 4: H₃CHC=CH and H on top; H and C₂H₅ on bottom of C=C]

Question 9

When considering the H and Cl bonded to C-2, Cl has a higher atomic mass than H and therefore is of higher priority. Similarly out of Cl and I, I has a higher priority. Both the higher priority groups are on the opposite side of the plane. So, the isomer is in the trans-position. The answer is B.

AMSAT Style Questions

Question (1-5).

Two or more, different compounds, which have the same molecular formula but different structural formula are called isomers and this phenomenon is known as isomerism. Structural isomerism basically occurs due to different arrangements of atoms within the molecule.

1. The pairs that represent structural isomerism are

A. $CH_3CH_2CH_2CH_2CH_2OH$ $H_3C-\underset{\underset{CH_3}{|}}{\overset{\overset{CH_3}{|}}{C}}-CH_2OH$

B. $HO-\bigcirc-OCH_3$ $H_3CO-\bigcirc-OH$

C. $H_3C-\underset{\underset{OH}{|}}{CH}-CH_2-CH_3$ $H_3C-CH_2-\underset{\underset{OH}{|}}{CH}-CH_3$

D. $(CH_3)_3CCl$ $H_3C-\underset{\underset{CH_3}{|}}{\overset{\overset{Cl}{|}}{C}}-CH_3$

2. The pairs that represent the same compound are:

A. 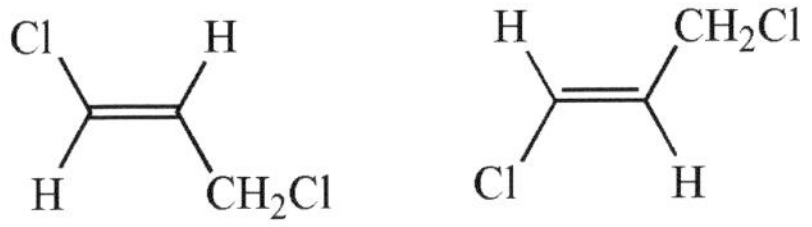
![structures]

B.

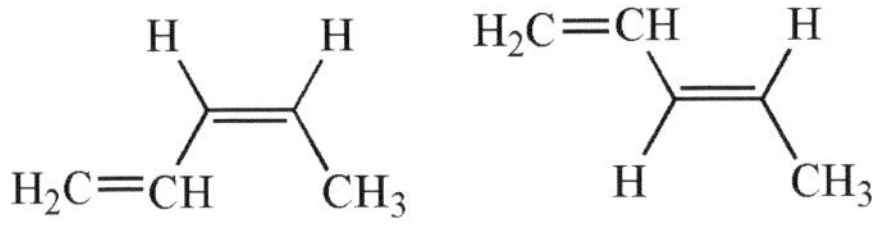

C.

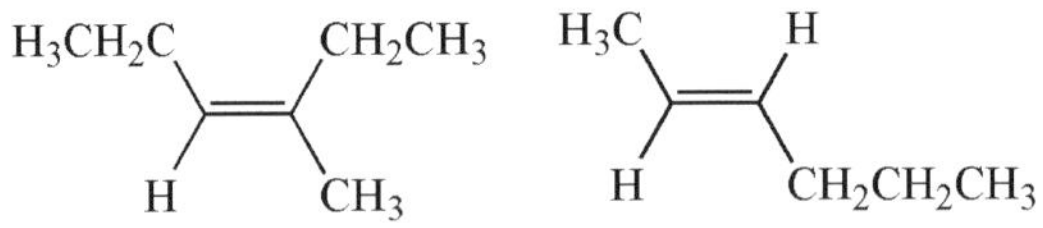

D. None of these

Question 3.

In nature, certain scents come from isomers of the same molecule. One example of this is the carvone molecule. A change in the conformation of this molecule results in two distinctly different scents as shown:

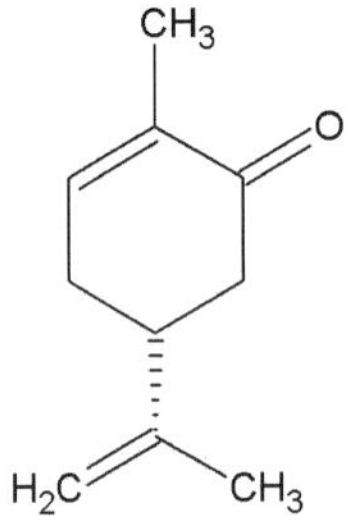

Spearmint 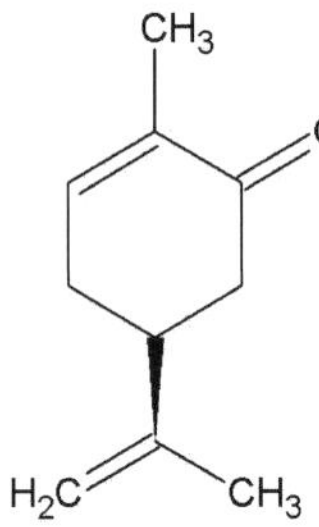   Caraway Seed

3. These types of isomers are known as
   A. structural isomers
   B. geometrical isomers
   C. chain isomers
   D. optical isomers

Question 4.

In stereoisomerisms, the atoms making up the isomers are joined up in the same order, but still have different spatial arrangements. Geometric isomerism is one form of stereoisomerisms. Geometric isomers will take either the cis- or trans- configuration.

I.

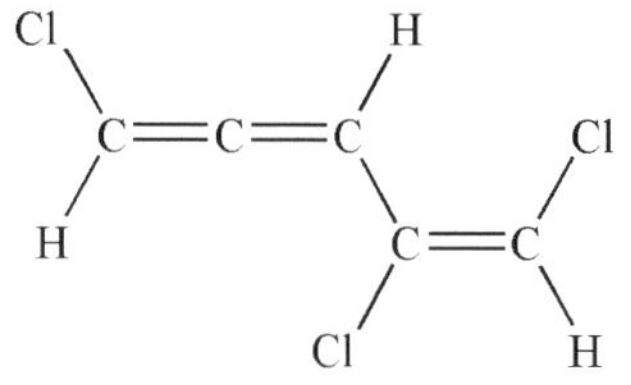

$$\begin{array}{c}ClH\\ C=C=C\\ HCl\end{array}$$

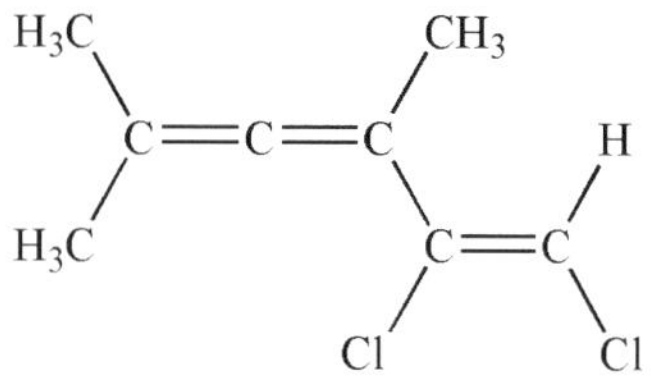

II.

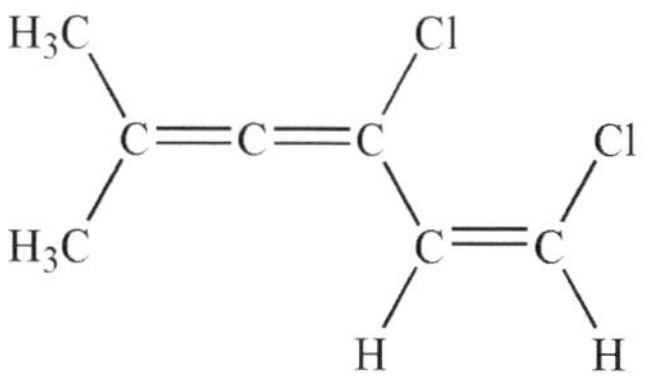

$$\begin{array}{c}H_3CCl\\ C=C=C\\ H_3CCl\end{array}$$

III.

$$\begin{array}{c}H_3CCH_3\\ C=C=C\\ H_3CH\end{array}$$

IV.

$$\begin{array}{c}ClH\\ C=C=C\\ H_3CCl\end{array}$$

(with additional C=C groups as shown)

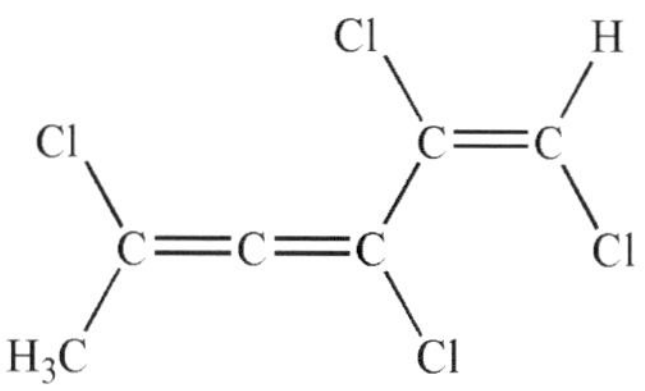

4. Which of the following molecules are present in the trans-configuration?
   A. I and III
   B. II and III
   C. I and IV
   D. III and IV

Question 5.

Hydrogenation reactions are exothermic reaction.

5. The most stable among the following alkenes is,

	Alkene	H (hydrogenation) in KJ mol-1
A. cis	$CH_3CH = CHCH_3$	-120
B.	$CH_3CH_2CH = CH_2$	-127
C. trans	$CH_3CH = CHCH_3$	-115
D.	$CH_3CH = CH_2$	-126

Question (6-10).

A carbon atom that is bonded to four different groups is called an asymmetric carbon. Optical isomers contain an asymmetric carbon atom in their molecules which allows the molecule to have two forms and for the compound to be optically active.

6. Which of the following have an asymmetric carbon atom?

A.
$$\begin{array}{c} \text{Cl} \;\; \text{Br} \\ | \;\;\; | \\ \text{H}-\text{C}-\text{C}-\text{H} \\ | \;\;\; | \\ \text{H} \;\;\; \text{H} \end{array}$$

B.
$$\begin{array}{c} \text{H} \;\; \text{Cl} \\ | \;\;\; | \\ \text{H}-\text{C}-\text{C}-\text{Cl} \\ | \;\;\; | \\ \text{H} \;\;\; \text{H} \end{array}$$

C.
$$\begin{array}{c} \text{H} \;\; \text{Cl} \\ | \;\;\; | \\ \text{H}-\text{C}-\text{C}-\text{D} \\ | \;\;\; | \\ \text{H} \;\;\; \text{Cl} \end{array}$$

D.
$$\begin{array}{c} \text{H} \;\; \text{H} \\ | \;\;\; | \\ \text{H}-\text{C}-\text{C}-\text{CH}_3 \\ | \;\;\; | \\ \text{Br} \;\; \text{OH} \end{array}$$

7. Each of the following compounds are expected to be optically active except:

A.
$$\begin{array}{c} \text{H} \\ | \\ \text{HO}-\text{C}-\text{COOH} \\ | \\ \text{CH}_3 \end{array}$$

B. $CH_3CH{=}CH{-}CH(OH){-}CHO$

C.
$$\begin{array}{c} \text{CH}_3 \\ | \\ \text{H}_3\text{C}-\text{C}-\text{OOCH}_3 \\ | \\ \text{H} \end{array}$$

D. None of the above

Question (8-11).

Any object that cannot be superimposed on its mirror image is said to be chiral. A chiral molecule cannot be superimposed on its mirror image; the molecule and its mirror image molecule are different compounds and represent a pair of stereoisomerisms called enantiomers. A compound that is not optically inactive (absence of chiral carbon) does not rotate the plane of polarized light.

8. Which of the following compounds can exist as a pair of enantiomers?

A. CH₃CHCl₂

B. 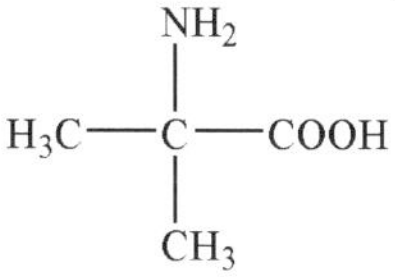 H₃C—C(NH₂)(CH₃)—COOH

C. H₂N—C(CH₂OH)(H)—CH₃

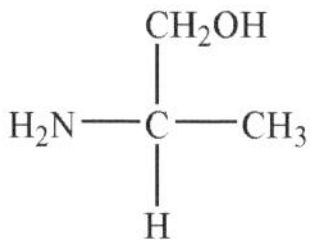

D. F—CH₂—COOH

9. Which of the following compound does not rotate the plane of polarized light?

A. 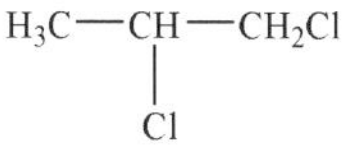 H₃C—CH(Cl)—CH₂Cl

B. H₃C—CH₂—C(Br)(I)—CH₂Br

C. H₂N—CH₂—COOH

D. 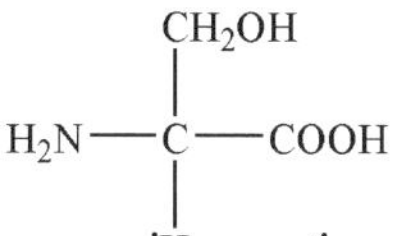 H₂N—C(CH₂OH)—COOH

10. Which of the following compounds can occur in enantiomeric form?

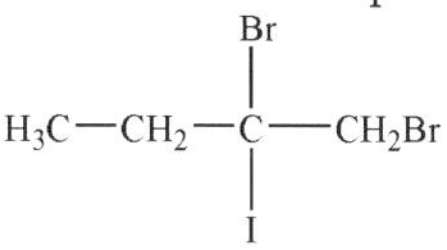

A. 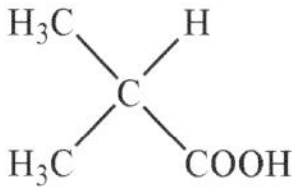 H₃C, H₃C, H, COOH on central C

B. 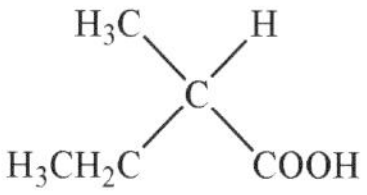 H₃C, H₃CH₂C, H, COOH on central C

C. H₃C, H, H, COOH on central C

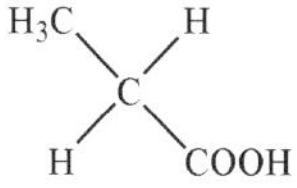

D. 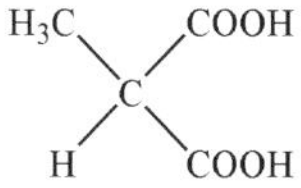 H₃C, H, COOH, COOH on central C

11. How many optically active forms are possible for a compound with the following chemical formula

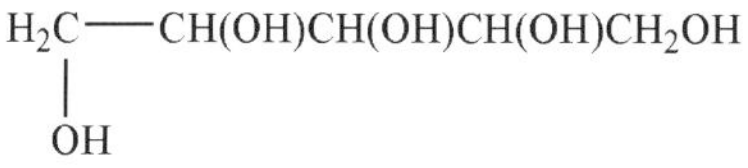

H₂C—CH(OH)CH(OH)CH(OH)CH₂OH
|
OH

A. 2
B. 3
C. 4
D. 8

Solution

Note: Use your own 3-step method

Question 1.
Only the structures given in answer A are structural isomers as the order of arrangement of carbon atoms is different. The other three pairs are the same compound. The compounds given in answer A are chain isomers.

Question 2.
The pair given in answer A represents the same compound, since the order of arrangement of carbon atoms and position of the double bond are the same, and both are trans isomers. The pair given in answer B is a pair geometrical isomer whereas in C, the position of the double bond is different.

Question 3.
STEP 1 = > What do you need to determine to solve the problem?
You need to figure out what type of isomers are represented by the chemical structures given

STEP 2 = > What relevant data provided in this problem is necessary in order to answer the question?
Two chemical structures are given, with only one subtle difference between the structures, the first has the bond coming off of the ring structure going into the plane of the paper and the other has the bond coming out of the plane of the paper.

STEP 3 = > Use the relevant data to solve the question
To solve this problem, you need to recognize the difference in the structure of the two molecules given and then draw on some general knowledge of isomers you have learned. Answers A and C are basically the same, a chain isomer is a form of a structural isomer and these occur when the carbon skeleton is the same but the functional groups are in different positions. This is not the case with our compounds. Our compounds are stereoisomers. Recall that geometric isomers require a double bond, and the conformational change occurs around the double bond to give either the cis or trans configuration, again not the case with our compounds, so B is incorrect. The correct answer is D; optical isomers. Optical isomers require a chiral or asymmetric carbon centre. The bond where the difference in conformation occurs is about a carbon with 4 different groups attached (a chiral centre).

Question 4.
STEP 1 = > What do you need to determine to solve the problem?
You need to determine which structures are in the trans configuration.

STEP 2 = > What relevant data provided in this problem is necessary in order to answer the question?
The structures of the molecules to be analyzed are provided. All of these molecules display two different alkene bonds about which configurational differences can occur. You will also need to recall that cis- means same side and trans- means across.

STEP 3 = > Use the relevant data to solve the question
In molecule I, two Cl atoms lie across from each other within one of the double bonds, and the Cl and large side group lie across from each other in the other set of double bonds, so it has the trans-configuration. In molecule II, one of the double bonds has the Cl and large side group on the same side of the molecule (cis-), and the other part of the molecule can take neither the cis or trans-configuration since it has two methyl groups on the same end of the molecule. In molecule III, similar to molecule, there are two methyl groups on the same end of one section of the molecule, so it can take neither the cis- or trans-configuration. The other double bond within the molecule has two Cl groups on the same side of the molecule and thus is in the cis-configuration. Molecule IV has Cl groups across from each other in both sets of double bonds so it is also taking the trans-configuration. Therefore, the correct answer is C.

Note: Try the rest of the solutions by writing out your own 3-step method.

Question 5.
Since hydrogenation is exothermic, the smaller the ΔH is (numerically, i.e. absolute value), the more stable the alkene will be relative to its parent alkane. The answer is C. Smallest $|\Delta H|$ value.

Question 6.
A carbon atom that is bonded to four different groups is called an asymmetric carbon. The compound given in answer D contains a chiral or asymmetric carbon.

$$H-\underset{Br}{\overset{H}{C}}-\underset{OH}{\overset{H}{\overset{*}{C}}}-CH_3$$

Question 7.
Only Methyl-2-methyl propanoate does not contain a chiral carbon, so it is optically inactive. The answer is C.

$$H_3C-\underset{\underset{H}{|}}{\overset{\overset{CH_3}{|}}{C}}-OOCH_3$$

Note the absence of a chiral carbon.
This question is a typical question where your knowledge will act as a boost. Though knowledge is not measured here, you can do it very fast, if you are highly familiar with the concept.

Question 8.
The optical isomers, which are mirror images of each other, are called enantiomers. The compound containing a chiral carbon (a carbon with four different attached side groups) exists as a pair of enantiomers. The answer is C.

Question 9.
A compound that is optically inactive (absence of chiral carbon) does not rotate the plane of polarized light. The only compound that does not have a chiral carbon is answer C, there are two H side groups. So, this compound is optically inactive and will have no effect on the plane polarized light.

Question 10.
The compound given in answer B contains a chiral carbon and therefore can occur in enantiomeric form.

$$H_3CH_2C-\underset{CH_3}{\overset{COOH}{|}}-H \qquad \bigg| \qquad H-\underset{CH_3}{\overset{COOH}{|}}-CH_2CH_3$$

Question 11.
The number of optically active isomers = 2^n
Where n is the number of chiral carbon atoms
These are three chiral carbon atoms, so the compound exists in $2^3=8$ optically active forms. The correct answer is D.

Printed in Great Britain
by Amazon